SAVED

Overcoming a 45-Year Gambling Addiction

PETER AND STEPH SHILTON

AD LIB

First published in 2021 by Ad Lib Publishers Ltd
15 Church Road
London, SW13 9HE

www.adlibpublishers.com

Text © 2021 Peter and Steph Shilton

Hardback ISBN 978-1-913543-64-8
eBook ISBN 978-1-913543-63-1

A CIP catalogue record for this book is available
from the British Library.

Printed in the UK

10 9 8 7 6 5 4 3 2 1

How love saved the England football legend from
a 45-year gambling addiction

A book of two halves – from two sides of the story

"The UK is entering into a gambling epidemic."
Peter Shilton

ACKNOWLEDGEMENTS

Special thanks to all those at Ad Lib publishing: Jon Rippon, John Blake, Robert Nichols and Martin Palmer, plus our ghost writers, Harry Harris and Linda Udall.

We are grateful for support from Gary Lineker OBE, Jon Holmes Media, Charles Ritchie, Carolyn Harris MP, the Rt. Hon Sir Iain Duncan Smith MP, Matt Gaskell, the Leeds & York Partnership NHS Foundation Trust, Stewart Kenny, co-founder of Paddy Power, Brian Chappell and Justice for Punters.

Thanks also to Fatal Attraction Hairdressers, Colchester; Paul Cudmore, Proshoot Photography, Colchester; and Paul Millsom, LeTalbooth, Dedham.

We'd like to dedicate our book to:

Les Shilton (Peter's Father) & Natalie Cooke (Steph's Daughter, Missy)

And in memory of

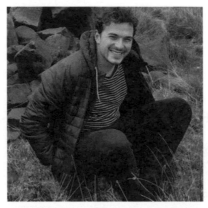

Jack Ritchie (28/12/1992 – 22/11/2017)

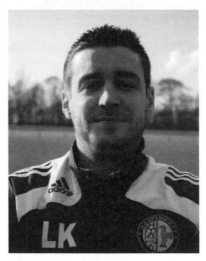

Lewis Keogh (15/10/1979 – 01/11/2013)

All of these individuals inspired us to tell our story.

CONTENTS

FOREWORD

GARY LINEKER, OBE

I was seven years old when my dad and grandad took me to Filbert Street for the first time. That first walk up the stairs. That first sight of the terraces. That first smell of professional football. That first glimpse of the hallowed green rectangle. It was unforgettable. It was thrilling. It was magical. All enhanced by the fact that the visitors were Manchester United. The United of Best, Charlton and Law. But it was not the Holy Trinity that caught this young man's eye that day. It was the Leicester goalkeeper. My dad told me he was a local lad like me. I was transfixed. He was incredible. He had such extraordinary agility and made save after save. I told my dad I wanted to be a goalkeeper – a goalkeeper like Peter Shilton.

Of course, that did not happen, but whenever I played with my younger brother, Wayne, in the garden, I was always in goal. I soon realised that I would not be big enough to be between the sticks and eventually ended up disliking goalkeepers. They all too often got in the way. I never disliked Peter Shilton, though, he was my boyhood hero. I was heartbroken when he left Leicester around my fourteenth birthday. Little did I know that some ten years later, I would be sharing a room with the great man whilst on England duty.

We were roommates for six years, two Leicester lads living their dreams. Shilts (yes, he had become Shilts to me at that point) retired from international football after the World Cup in Italy in 1990 as the most capped English player in history.

We had a wonderful friendship, with the odd hilarious moment. Shilts will recall us attempting to make a film in Mexico during the 1986

World Cup for ITV. I was to serve him some afternoon tea on a silver platter. The joke being that I was the goalie's lackey (yes, he was the goalie on my team now) and therefore did what he asked, which was largely true. Filming started and I hid in the bathroom ready to come out with my platter and pour his tea. It took us about a hundred takes. Every time I sneaked out of the bathroom we burst into laughter. We just could not do it without one or both of us giggling.

And then there was the time we got shafted by the rest of the England squad at Italia '90. To keep everyone occupied and to alleviate boredom (there were no mobile phones, no internet and no computer games back then) we did various activities. One that was very popular was race nights. Fred Street, the England physio at the time, had tapes of old race meetings from various parts of the world. Peter and I were the bookies, imaginatively called 'Honest Shilts and Links'. I had had some experience of running a book and, as bookmakers do, we made sure that we were well in front. Then came the sting. Fred allowed Gazza to see the result of the last race. Everyone placed their bets on a number of horses. The big hitters, though, were waiting for the odds to drift out on the horse they *knew* would win. Eventually, when the odds were around ten to one, in they came. Big bet after big bet was placed. Shilts and I looked at each other and feared the worst. Not even Peter Shilton could save this one. As the winner crossed the finishing line the entire squad were doing the conga around the swimming pool in celebration.

The remarkable aspect of Shilts' remarkable contribution to football is not just his obvious brilliance, or the many trophies he won, but the longevity of his career. I'd watched him most weeks since I was seven and yet, when I retired from playing the game, Shilts was still playing. In total, he notched up an extraordinary one thousand league games.

This book, I know, is not just about his football career, but other more serious matters. I was aware that Shilts loved a bet – how could I not be? Quite frequently when we were visiting he would ask me to leave the room as he wanted to put his horse racing bets on privately. Later, I found out that gambling had become problem for him. And that it had cost him an awful lot.

I am delighted that Shilts has addressed his addiction and is now raising awareness of the dangers of gambling. There has never been a more important time to shine a light on the dark side of betting. Football is awash with bookmakers' adverts and sponsorships and they suck people into a world that can lead to misery and desperation. It's deeply concerning. So this book is a most welcome contribution to the efforts to highlight the perils of gambling. I am as proud of Peter Shilton now as I was on that first day at Filbert Street. Well played, goalie.

INTRODUCTION

In this powerful memoir, Peter Shilton, England's record cap holder, opens his heart and reveals how his 45-year addiction to gambling nearly destroyed him and how the love and support of his wife, Steph, enabled him to turn his life around and defeat his demons. This is the story of how he was saved – how he saved himself, and how Steph's love saved him.

Peter admits to his self-destructive obsession with gambling and tells the inspiring story of how he was able to overcome his secret and silent addiction. It is a book that offers hope for others suffering or heading along the same downward spiral. Peter found himself again and discovered how to beat his dark addiction. Steph, formerly an NHS Manager for more than 20 years, knows that as the wife of an addict she can help raise awareness in several public health areas. She now wants to reach out to anyone affected by a partner's gambling to help them too. For the first time, the wife of one of football's greatest ever players, tells her side of the story. This book is as much about Steph as it is about Peter. It's a story of chronic addiction seen from both sides but with an uplifting ending. Steph offers advice to the loved ones of people struggling with addiction and reveals how she worked tirelessly to help Peter tackle his.

The book is also about the Shiltons' campaign and their work with the government and the charity Gambling with Lives in the battle to prevent the scourge of suicides associated with gambling addictions as well as the associated mental health issues. *Saved* has a distinct purpose – to highlight the dangers of gambling when it becomes an addiction not just in the privileged world of football but in all walks of life. The Shiltons want to confront football's unhealthy relationship with gambling. The game's establishment takes tens of millions of pounds from the gambling industry in the form of advertising revenue and sponsorship fees. It's time to address the issue and make a real change.

PROLOGUE

PETE'S STORY

There I stood, aged about nine, with my mum and younger brother, looking up and watching my dad charging towards us at the fairground, waving his hands high in the air, his face beaming with excitement. "I've won!" he said. We had the joy of being on holiday in Mablethorpe and the fun of all the rides at the fairground, and now we were an ecstatic little family celebrating dad's lucky spell on the horses. Ironically, at the time of his win, I was in the arcade.

Did this moment sow the seeds in me that pushed me to be forever chasing that big win? Why not? Winning ran through my every vein for as long as I can remember. I possessed the goal on the football pitch. Standing between the posts, evaluating the opponents, studying their performance, the goal it belonged to me. Within minutes I could weigh the danger of any player on the pitch, protecting my area like a wild predator. "Come on, try and beat me" was etched my entire mind as I dominated my area. I was on guard, every inch of my body and mind was on high alert. I could never be beaten. I had to win. Every shot thrown at me, I countered with determination and intensity. I had to succeed – winning was crucial to my very existence. From when I was very young I was always obsessed in my art of goalkeeping and fixated on never losing a match.

A million miles away from my professional world lay a dark and lonely place. This world crept up on me very gradually. I guess it started as a hobby, but it grew into yet another obsession – only this one would most certainly end badly. It would cost me almost everything. I eventually ended up living in a nightmare which cruelly overtook my entire life and well-being – like a disease spreading through me. With the continued desire to win driving me, I felt I couldn't go any lower. The reality of not winning began shadowing my thoughts. All this was happening as I welcomed a wonderful new lady to my life. Not only did I think she was beautiful, but she was such wonderful company and great fun to be with – I was totally in love with her. In my heart, I knew that my need to win and beat the bookie meant that I ran the risk of losing the love of my life. And so an agonising tug of war began…

STEPH'S STORY

As I walked along the long, carpeted corridor towards the lifts I looked out of the windows to see the floodlit site of a golf course. Being a keen golfer, I had a pang of regret at not having packed my beloved golf clubs. I had to remind myself I was there to relax and sing. As I approached the lift doors, they opened and there stood an older gentleman. Little did I know that very second had sealed my fate, because there stood the man who I was about to go an incredible journey with and be with for the rest of my life. I was about to enter into a complete overhaul of the world I knew but I would also be stepping into a dark world which had the potential to destroy us both.

Further along our timeline together I found myself walking along another long corridor. This one didn't have a plush carpet but pictures of what looked like football legends decorated the walls. As I held Pete's hand, guiding me down the busy tunnel, I noticed a prominent picture of Pete plastered all over part of the corridor wall. My jaw must have hit the floor as I froze and exclaimed, "That's you!" He laughed and responded, "Yes, Steph, I told you I had played a bit in my time." With my head in a whirl, walking briskly and hand-in-hand with Pete and the FA officials at Wembley stadium, I found myself at the end of the dark tunnel standing in the stadium with Wembley's pitch in front of me, surrounded by 90,000 chanting football fans. Never had I experienced such enormity; the sound alone was overwhelming. My heart was literally pounding. As I turned back to look into the tunnel the entire England squad were all lined up, charged and ready to run onto the greatest football pitch in England. The team all nodded in respect to Pete as, one by one, they made their way into their arena. My first experience of the football world and here I was. The small bubble I had lived in had just burst forever. Life, as I knew it, would now never be the same – everything had changed.

But my new bubble would burst one sunny August day just a few years on. The postman arrived with a bundle of letters. Whilst checking through them, I noticed a bank statement addressed to Pete. He was working in India, thousands upon thousands of miles away from me, and there I sat with his bank statement sealed in an envelope now in my hands. For three days I repeatedly picked it up from the mantlepiece where I had placed it. I kept holding it, telling myself I should open it. I knew that finally this envelope would reveal the truth to me. It held all of the answers of months and months of anxious questions. Here in one white envelope lay my future but also my deepest fears. Finally, after agonising with myself and terrified that my worst concerns might be true, with shaking hands I nervously sat alone in our quiet home and slowly opened the envelope. I knew it was wrong – it was such an intrusion on my beloved Pete but in my mind I knew it was the right thing to do. There in front of me lay the answers in factual black and white, page after page…

THE FIRST HALF

OUR MESSAGE OF HOPE

The reason for writing this book is to deliver a message, through these pages, to those suffering due to gambling addiction – do not despair, there is a way out and support is at hand. We are here; ready to support and understand. We are not qualified counsellors but we are highly qualified in living through the experience of gambling addiction.

We intend this to be a self-help book, not just for elite sportsmen, but also for every ordinary person out there who finds themselves hooked on gambling. We wrote this book for the gambling addict, to help them realise and appreciate there is a way out of their seemingly never-ending nightmare and that it is possible to turn your life around. It is also for those loved ones close to the addict. We want to support the partners, brothers, sisters, mothers, fathers and friends of gambling addicts who suffer such torment and give them tools to help them with their life change by finding a way out for the gambling addict. It's also intended to educate everybody about the perils of gambling and gambling addiction.

We are not anti-gambling. Gambling sensibly, moderately and for fun is fine. It can be a form of relaxation and an acceptable hobby, providing it is within your means and in moderation. Having a bet, for a stake you can afford, now and again, is perfectly fine and good fun. There are many who *can* bet reasonably and within their limits. However, regrettably more and more are betting *outside* of their limits. Trust us, we know how that can happen. When it gets out of hand, it can be life changing, debilitating, financially crippling and can, in some cases, lead to extreme actions like suicide.

1

Gambling is becoming an epidemic – it is an illness, a disease, and needs to be recognised as such. It is an addiction, just like alcohol or drug addiction, there is no difference. You could say it's actually much worse because it is so hidden, so secretive – if someone is hooked on alcohol or drugs you can often see it, it's evident in the way they walk, talk or the way they look. But gambling is much more clandestine. Betting beyond your means can lead to real crisis and much, much worse.

We are writing as a victim of gambling addiction for 45 years, and as a partner who subsequently became a victim. So we know that there is a feeling of loneliness, isolation and hopelessness. But there *is* hope, and we believe that this book will be the start of the process that an addict needs to begin in order to come through it. The time is right to open up about the real extent of the damage this addiction can have but it's also time to shine a light on how there is a way through it.

For both of us, many a tear has been shed while discussing the situation from both sides – the addict, and the addict's partner. It's been truly a game of two halves to work together to tell the story of the thing that had eaten into our lives for so many years.

It has been tough unburdening the truth but extremely cathartic. It has equally been a relief – almost a form of counselling – for both of us, to get everything off our chests, confront the demons and the staggering losses with the online bookie, to experience the realisation and then the redemption. It is said that love conquers all, well, it conquered the 45-year gambling addiction of a man who had squandered almost all his entire lifetime's achievements and fortune without really knowing he was doing it.

Like any addict, be it to drugs or alcohol, the final cut-off point, or the tipping point, was the hardest of all. The decision to quit; then, when you say it, to mean it. That was six years ago and since then not a single penny has been squandered with the bookies, and we have never been happier. For us this is also a love story: the chance meeting in a lift; how we fell in love; our white wedding; our idyllic, romantic honeymoon. There will be some football, some funny stories and some inside track within these pages, but that is about all. This book is something completely different to memoirs that have come before because it has a purpose, a vision and an important message – a potentially life-saving message.

2

We want change. No, we *demand* change, and we are campaigning vigorously for change.

There will be the average punter who likes a bet now and again, it's a hobby, a relaxation for a lot of people, they love to go to the races, and they bet within their limits. They might even be too tight to spend too much! But the very nature of gambling is that it can become addictive and compulsive and, for many, can do so all too easily. With online betting you can be sitting on the beach, pick up your phone, and gamble. You can be just about anywhere and gamble. The issue is not how much you gamble, how often, but if you can afford to gamble.

We are working with people who can facilitate change to discuss helping to tackle the menace of gambling including Carolyn Harris MP, the Chair of the All-Party Parliamentary Group on Gambling-Related Harm. We are also working with the charity Gambling with Lives, which was set up by the bereaved parents of gamblers.

Whilst the betting companies see their profits soaring, many of their customers are finding themselves in misery and trapped in a compulsive betting snare. More and more lives will be ruined, there will be more and more suicides, a whole new generation of children caught in the betting trap, more families devastated – unless there are adequate regulations brought in and quickly. Gambling is a hugely profitable industry. The companies have recently made moves to ensure clients' safety and well-being but much of this is largely public relations. The key aim is to make as much money as possible. They might say safeguards are in place but, clearly, they don't go far enough, clearly they are not working well enough. There needs to be more, much more. How many lives will be lost before real, effective action is taken? How can it be good enough when pop-up adverts, free spins of the wheel, free bets and other such aggressive advertising is still being sent to vulnerable and addictive gamblers. How can the industry be taking responsibility when more and more ill-protected youngsters are committing suicide. All this at the same time as measures are taken so they either close down or curtail their stakes on accounts that might be on a winning streak.

The epidemic is with us right now and the knock-on effect is that it will put extra strain on the NHS and our already stretched mental health resources. There will be more patients needing treatment for depression and much worse. We all know the consequences of drug taking, alcohol abuse, excessive smoking but gambling seems to still be under the radar for the medical consequences it is causing.

The betting industry needs to be held to account. There needs to be much greater safeguards, less self-interest and less focus on the huge amounts of revenue the gambling industry brings into the government. For so many years there was a reluctance to highlight the dangers of smoking and introduce curbs on the advertising of cigarettes, place warning notices on the packages and then ban smoking in indoor public spaces. How long did it take to persuade the government to enforce these measures? Too long. It's now the same with gambling. There is too much advertising and it's often too aggressive. In this aspect, football has to be held accountable too as there is far too much sponsorship from the gambling industry. Far too many team shirts are advertising and pushing gambling on the football fans many of whom are children.

Children are getting hooked on gambling very easily. We were appalled to learn the story of a teenager who took his own life because he was hooked on gambling at the age of just seventeen. Children love their smartphones and on those they can gamble whenever and wherever they might be. Vulnerable children are prone to take up gambling. In July 2020, a House of Lords report estimated that around 55,000 children have a gambling habit that is out of control right now in the UK and it's getting worse. There needs to be more education in schools about this problem.

So, this is our story but it's also a call for understanding and change. We met, fell in love and after that we faced our greatest challenge. The old cliché is true, love *does* conquer all. We want this book to show the thousands if not millions of people currently hooked on gambling that there is a way out and we can help you find it.

CHAPTER 1

UPLIFTING!

PETE'S STORY

It was a chance encounter at an event that changed my life completely. I was booked as a guest speaker at the lavish Stoke by Nayland Hotel, Golf & Spa that is idyllically located in the Dedham Vale area of outstanding natural beauty, in the countryside just outside of Colchester. It must have been fate, as it was here that I met Steph – my own 'natural beauty' – purely by chance! It was to be a life changing encounter.

I was speaking at a Rotary Club dinner taking place at the hotel. I had another personal appearance commitment the following day – ironically, opening a Corals betting shop in Kent – so I was determined to have an early night and make an early getaway the next morning. This is why fate played such a hand here. Normally, I like to drive home after a long evening working as a guest speaker. I would normally be driving back in the early hours when the traffic is light and the roads are clearer, with the adrenalin still kicking in from the personal appearance. But this time, due to the personal appearance scheduled the next day, I opted to take up the offer of the overnight stay. It was rare I stayed overnight and, even though I was living on my own, it was usually my preference to go back home.

I was all dressed up looking like James Bond – well, I wish – in my dickie bow tie and tuxedo. Whenever I am on duty as a guest speaker, I am aware that people at the event want a memento of the evening and so, as usual, I was carrying a wallet of photographs that I could easily sign and distribute. I was going down in the lift when the door opened and in stepped Steph with some girlfriends. Next thing, I'm there standing next to Steph. She looked stunning, gorgeous. And you know that instant feeling that there is some sort of connection? I felt it, especially when she made me laugh when she asked: "Are you a musician?" I discovered later that Steph was a jazz singer, and that there was also a music convention at the hotel, which was the reason why Steph and her friends were spending a couple of nights at the venue as part of a girls' spa break.

"No," I replied, "I'm a speaker."

"What are you speaking about?"

"I'm speaking about football."

It was hugely refreshing that Steph didn't know who I was and had no idea why anyone would be talking about football at a hotel.

Later, after the dinner, I was chatting with the organiser, and enjoying a glass of red wine as I was not driving home that night. My plan was to finish my drink and get off to bed. But the organiser was very agreeable and persuaded me to allow him to top up my glass. I had just put my head in the large restaurant bar to see if there was any sport on the TV when I spotted Steph sitting there on her own, whilst her friends mingled.

"Hello," said Steph, when she spotted me, "would you like to join me?"

There was a group of golfers in the corner of the bar, and it was clear they knew who I was, even though Steph was still very much in the dark. I don't know if her friends had recognised me. Probably not.

As the evening wore on I discovered Steph was a singer, and that people had been waiting for her to perform and were encouraging her to come up to sing. Later, Steph told me that she wouldn't normally have been keen to get up and sing, but she confessed that she wanted to because she wanted to impress me. The song she chose was "Mr Bojangles". When she finished she got a lovely round of applause from everybody in the bar – including me.

Someone shouted: "Go on, Peter, help her off the stool!" And then one of the golfers called out: "Don't drop her, Peter!" and his group of golfing pals laughed. I am pretty sure Steph still didn't have an inkling about who I was and must have been wondering what all that was about, but she still laughed at the banter in the room.

Later, while we were chatting away, Steph became inquisitive about my wallet of photographs and she asked: "What's in there?" I told her it was filled with photos of myself. We had a few drinks and at the end of the night we exchanged numbers. Before we said goodnight that evening, I reached down, handed one of the pictures to her and told her that I used to play a bit of football. I still don't think she was any the wiser.

Well, that was it really, that was our first meeting. Maybe, if I hadn't had my glass filled and been persuaded to have one last glass of red in the bar, I would have probably gone to bed happily enough and not gone to the restaurant bar. Then again, if Steph hadn't walked into that lift, she wouldn't have walked into my life. It was as if somebody up there was determined to throw us together. It was definitely fate that brought us together. We immediately got on well. I thought she had such a great personality and there was clearly something that clicked between us – there was a chemistry, you could tell.

It was always my intention to contact her and to see if it led to anything. What did I have to lose? Not long afterwards, I texted her suggesting that it would be great if I could see her again. I lived on my own at the time and I used to pop along to my local – a lovely olde worlde pub – a couple of times a week to have a pint of Guinness, some fish and chips and study the *Racing Post*. Instead of reading the paper, I started using this time to text Steph. I began chatting to her and we were laughing and smiling all the time. The two lovely elderly waitresses, used to seeing me on my own studying my newspaper, must have noticed I was on my phone and wondered what I was up to. They kept smiling at me and I could tell they were thinking: 'What's going on? He's up to something. He must be on the phone to a lady.' Well, that's exactly what was going on – that was me arranging our first proper date!

STEPH'S STORY

It's amazing how your whole life can change in just one moment. A chance meeting can lead to lasting love and that's what happened for me and Pete. The moment I set eyes on him I just knew we'd be together, and our love story started right there in that lift!

It was in February 2012 and I was away with a group of girlfriends for a weekend break at a lovely hotel and spa in the countryside just outside of Colchester. I had been single for a long time and my daughter, Missy, had always been my priority. We had just welcomed a beautiful granddaughter, Summer into the family and Missy was settled with her partner, Dean. I knew their relationship was completely solid and

I knew they would have a long, secure future together and a beautiful little family. So I knew that, for the first time in years, it was my time to move on. Having hit my early 40s I felt able to do things for myself for the first time in years. I thought I might start travelling more and even felt I would be open to a lasting relationship. I knew I wanted to meet someone on my travels.

I was a focused career woman working as a manager in the NHS. I could support myself as I had a good income. I was very serious about my career and have always had a strong work ethic but there is another side of my personality – the singer and performer. When I sang it could appear that I was always happy and bubbly and having a great time. I loved what I was doing but often that would be a front. I had good friends and loved a night out but deep down I was actually lonely and realised that I had been for such a long time.

I told Missy that I was at a point in my life when I felt ready to see more of the world and I wanted to start travelling and that, deep down, I hoped that I would meet someone on my travels and someone I was willing to commit to. At last, at 43 years old I was ready to start a new chapter in my life and I really felt that I wanted some excitement.

Despite working full time, I still found time to relax and one of those occasions was that weekend away with some girlfriends. There was a jazz weekend on at the hotel with an open mic jamming session. I was really looking forward to having the chance to sing as well as having some relaxing 'me time' with the girls in the spa as we had booked in quite a few treatments.

On the Friday evening the girls and I booked into the hotel and made reservations in the restaurant. We got ready and were all in a really good mood. When the doors to the lift opened on our floor we all piled into the small lift. Being the smallest amongst them, I was squashed in and pressed right up against this really good-looking man who was tall and handsome. We were all giggling and all I could say to him was, "Hi, nice to meet you." He laughed as we were obviously all in a good mood and he came across as really nice. I was crammed right up against him.

He was wearing a tuxedo and I noticed that he had a small case with him which I thought had an instrument in it or music sheets, so I assumed he was with a band for the jazz night. I remember looking at his hands and noted that his fingers were slightly bent upwards. I wondered if he might be a pianist or a clarinet, trumpet or saxophone player. I said to him, "Are you with the jazz band? I'll be singing tonight so hopefully I'll see you there." He laughed and said that he wasn't a musician, but he would be speaking that evening. I thought that was really odd and asked him what he would be speaking about and when he said it was football I replied, "Oh, how dull." Of course, I had absolutely no idea who he was, and he just cracked up when I said that.

When we got out of the lift on the ground floor, he went his way and my friends and I went ours but not before I told him it was nice to meet him and he said, "Likewise." Although it was just a short lift ride I could tell there was chemistry between us. My girlfriends had been chatting and laughing amongst themselves but because Pete and I were pressed up against each other, facing each other, it had felt like we were in our own little bubble.

During dinner I kept thinking about him. I was sure he had been joking and winding me up and that he really was a musician because I couldn't imagine anyone doing a talk about football. Of course I realised that there were different functions going on in the hotel at the same time but, I have to admit, at that time I didn't even like football.

After dinner, my friends and I went to the main bar which was absolutely packed. Everyone was mingling and there was a great atmosphere in the room. At one point, I was sitting alone with a glass of wine, happily people watching. After a while, in walked Pete and he recognised me from our meeting in the lift. I was in a really good mood and it felt natural to say, "Oh, it's you again! Would you like to join me?" There was something intriguing about this man and I really wanted to find out more about him. The conversation just flowed.

We quickly established we were both single. There was no game-playing, we were completely honest. We talked non-stop and bells started to go off for me – could this person become someone very special? I was aware that he was a bit older than me – there was almost a 20-year difference between us and I wondered if that age gap might be a bit too much.

There was real banter between us, and it felt so relaxed and normal, like neither of us was trying too hard. I'm quite a private person but the two of us really opened up. We talked about our pasts and our feelings about life. It was as if we had known each other for ages. To be able to be so open and honest with a complete stranger made me realise that this could develop into something very special.

As we were chatting I asked him about his background and what he did, and he said, "I used to play a bit of football." It's hilarious to me now that, at the time, I had yet to find out what a legendary football star he really was. He totally played down his amazing career that first evening.

Looking back, although I didn't know how famous he was, he didn't once show off or keep talking about himself. I didn't feel that he was trying to impress me, he was just totally natural. He kept bringing the conversation back round to me and asking about my background and career. I made it clear that I was independent and took my work very seriously – so he knew I wasn't a 'dolly bird'. The bar was so busy, and we were engrossed in our conversation, but I still became aware of people looking at us. Especially the men who obviously knew who Pete was.

It was then time for me to take the mic. Although I can be quite shy and private I'm much more confident when I'm on stage. I sang the classic, "Mr Bojangles" which so many people love, and it was a hit with the audience. When I went to step down from the stool my friend turned to Pete and said, "Aren't you going to go and help her down?" There was a lot of hooting and laughter from the men who called out, "Don't drop her!" With hindsight, I realised they were joking about the fact that he was a famous goalkeeper. At the time I just laughed along. I thought he was so sweet, and I felt a true connection with this man. There was a lot of cheering, but I just thought the audience were showing appreciation of my voice.

Pete and I talked for hours. It was strange because I clearly remember that, when I stared into his eyes, I saw a real loneliness and he looked broken. We talked so much on that first night which was very rare in my experience, but it felt so *real*. We understood each other. We immediately clicked. I felt a genuine trust between us. We spoke about our feelings in a way that most people wouldn't do on a first encounter. We both revealed our vulnerable sides without any embarrassment which was so refreshing that it was astonishing.

At the end of the evening, he walked me to my room, kissed me in a very gentlemanly way and asked if he could get my number. At that point

I had butterflies and realised that I had thoroughly enjoyed his company and wanted to see him again.

The next morning my friends and I were on our way to have our spa treatments, so we were in the reception with our robes on when I bumped into Pete again as he was checking out. I suddenly felt a bit shy and awkward and that's when I knew I really liked him. He told me how lovely it was meeting me and that he'd like to take me out. He had definitely made an impression on me and despite the age difference there was a real attraction between us. He asked me what I was going to be doing that evening and I said, "The same as last night." Then he made me laugh by saying, "Well, don't have a drink with any strange men in the bar." Then he gave me his number and asked to me ring him before saying goodbye.

CHAPTER 2

THE FIRST DATE AND
NEW BEGINNINGS

PETE'S STORY

Steph suggested we stay at a hotel near Colchester. Years later, she would stay in that same hotel with her bridesmaids, ahead of our wedding. The hotel had a golf course and was set in a lovely location. I was really looking forward to the opportunity to get to know Steph much better after all our texting and chats on the phone.

Driving from my house in the Midlands, my mind was full of thoughts about where this was likely to go and how much I was looking forward to seeing Steph. I had a real feeling of optimism that this was a relationship that would prove to be long-lasting and something really special. We shared a connection and we also shared the fact that we were both at the stage in our lives where we needed a strong relationship. I must be honest, I felt lonely at this point in my life. I was living alone in the Midlands, waiting to sell the house after my divorce. Steph told me she hadn't had a relationship for a while either.

What didn't occur to me was whether it was fair to begin a relationship with Steph – or indeed anyone – when I had a problem I was hiding. In truth, I had no idea that I even had a problem at that stage. Why would I? Until it actually became undeniable that I was addicted – that it was an illness – and that, in reality, I urgently needed help, I was oblivious to it all. It never entered my head that this was something I needed to confront or share. With hindsight, that was exactly what I needed, and eventually, with Steph by my side, that's what I got. So that day, I was happy, excited and eagerly looking forward to seeing Steph again. It never crossed my mind that if, as I had hoped, the relationship developed, I would be burdening someone with my problems. I didn't see that I had a problem.

I had a steady income at the time, as well as my football pension – it was not as though gambling was going to leave me destitute. Only now can I see this was part of the problem, not just for me, but anyone who is in the grip of an addiction – especially gambling addiction. There are no obvious signs of a problem to outsiders, and the addict either doesn't know they have a problem or is in total denial about it. That was me.

As our relationship developed Steph learned that I liked a bet but had no clue to what extent until much further into our relationship. Until that moment, I didn't see how much it might impact on us. Until I sorted myself out, I honestly didn't realise that I had a problem.

We got on so well during that first date. We had a lovely meal at the hotel and quickly rekindled the feeling we had from the very first meeting in the lift and our chat in the bar the night we'd first met. It was just as we had both hoped. What struck me most about Steph was her sense of humour and her caring and strong personality. Her character suited me as I had a strong personality too and was clearly obsessive – you have to be to make your way to the top in football. While Steph was fun and good company, she also had a highly responsible job with the NHS. We quickly developed a good relationship. We were made for each other. The age difference never seemed to become an issue. I'd always been physically fit and in good shape, so I felt young for my age. Then again, Steph is young for her age too. But the difference in our ages wasn't a problem – in fact, I don't think it has ever even been discussed between us.

STEPH'S STORY

A couple of weeks after our first encounter we went on our first date. Peter and I had had a really lovely time together on the first night we met but I had sensed an unhappiness about him which I couldn't put my finger on. I was also a little bit worried about the age difference. I was getting a bit nervous about the idea.

Pete booked rooms for us at a really lovely hotel near Mersea Island that I'd recommended. He wanted us to be able to relax, have a few drinks and not rush home. On the day I was due to meet Pete for dinner I couldn't settle. I got all dressed up in a black dress and high heels in a bid to disguise my mere five foot one and a half inches height, then phoned Missy and said: "I can't do this, I'm going to have to cancel. He's really nice but I'm just too nervous." Thank goodness for Missy as she gave me the confidence to go for it. She said: "Mum, you can't back out of this. You can't do it to him. He's driven hundreds of miles to see you, you have to go and meet him. You'll be fine and you'll have a lovely time." She had a good vibe about it so that really helped me.

So, I phoned Pete. He was driving and answered on the car speaker. I was completely honest with him. I told him that I was feeling very nervous. Later, he said that he found my vulnerability very endearing but at the time he responded by saying that we were going to have a great time so I shouldn't worry.

I was waiting anxiously for him to arrive and started to think back to the first time we met. I remembered that he had been wearing a tuxedo that night. I had no idea what he was going to look like when he turned up. He insisted on coming to pick me up at my house and I was so relieved when I set eyes on him. He was just as handsome as I remembered. He was dressed casually but smartly in navy blue which really suited him, and I thought he was actually even more handsome than I remembered him. Also, he didn't look as old as I had remembered – in fact he looked younger. He gave me a kiss on the cheek, and I noticed that he was shaking a little and looked a bit nervous too. He admitted that he hadn't been on a date in years. From the start, we were both transparent about our insecurities.

When we arrived at the hotel we didn't check in straight away. Pete suggested we have a glass of wine in the bar which was a good way to calm our nerves. From that moment, we picked up where we left off. It was lovely. The conversation flowed and we couldn't stop laughing. It was obvious that we didn't take ourselves too seriously. Pete has since said that he liked the fact that, back then, I knew nothing about sport, or his famous background, and he thought it was great that he didn't have to talk about football all night.

Our first date was very much a secret as, being an NHS manager, I was used to keeping my private life very much away from my working life. They were totally separate, so only Missy and a close friend from the spa weekend knew about our date.

The bar was busy as the hotel is a popular golf resort and there were lots of men in there who had finished playing their rounds of golf. Pete suggested we move from the bar area into a quiet lounge. Unknown to me, at the time, he was trying to avoid being around fans. I thought he wanted to give all his attention to me, which I found quite endearing. He wanted to know all about my background and was especially interested in my career in the NHS. He really made a point of putting the focus on me and making me feel relaxed.

Dinner was booked for us in the main restaurant. We were greeted by the restaurant manager and taken to a beautiful, secluded table. It was very romantic, and I remember thinking; "Wow, this is amazing service." Over dinner we shared a bottle of champagne and I felt completely at ease with Pete, but I still had butterflies in my stomach which was a good sign. Being a semi-professional singer, I had plenty of confidence and could readily get up on a stage and sing and perform in front of lots of people. But it's a mask when you're putting on an act and performing. With my NHS job I had faced some heartbreaking situations and distressing scenes. You need to be strong, put on heavy armour and learn to build up inner strength in order to cope with those kind of things. But that night I suddenly felt completely exposed. I felt that the real me was coming out. I started telling Pete everything about myself and he did the same. Neither of us had ever done that in the past. I kept saying; "Oh my God, I've never told anyone about that before." I just trusted him implicitly. I had felt something special when we first met. We had connected on such a deep level and I was so happy that it was exactly the same the second time around. I knew we had something really good and I honestly felt, even after just two meetings, that it could become serious. We had the same sense of humour, the same outlook on life and similar beliefs. It was a real connection.

Although we talked openly and deeply we still had lots of light moments and fun and we were cracking up with laughter all through dinner. My work in the NHS was challenging so, in my personal life, I would just want to laugh and enjoy life to its full. At the end of the evening we got lost in the hotel trying to find our rooms, which made us both laugh. We've done that so many times now on trips we've been on together – we always tend to find the funny side of things.

The next day, before Pete took me home, we went for a drive as I wanted him to see some of the Essex coast. We went to Mersea Island, where we have now made our home, and Brightlingsea. Both are lovely places, and Pete was impressed with our coastline. We had a lovely lunch together but, after that, the mood was different and he seemed slightly sad. He dropped me home and it became clear that, after having had such a lovely time, we both felt deflated. We didn't want it to end. Pete said that Essex was really lovely and that he would like to come there more often, and I jokingly said: "You never know, you might end up falling in love with me and visiting more." He looked at me and smiled and said: "That just might happen." For the rest of the journey home we were both quiet.

We continued to phone and text each other daily that next week. I invited him to come and visit again the next weekend and stay at my home. From that point onwards, we both knew that we would be together and would spend the rest of our lives together.

When I first visited Pete's home in Warwickshire I asked him where his "football cups" were, expecting them to be on show. He laughed for ages at me. "What do you mean 'cups'?" he asked. I expected to see his 125 gold or silver England cups on show. He laughed and said, "They're *caps* – that you wear on your head." I looked at him, totally puzzled, and said, "I don't get it." I really didn't know anything about football. He was literally in hysterics. He hugged me and planted a kiss on the top of my head, still laughing.

Very soon we found ourselves missing each other more and more and it was becoming increasingly difficult being apart. Pete's visits to see me began to get longer and longer, sometimes staying three days in a row, then four and so on. Eventually we agreed together that life apart was miserable, and we were just counting down the hours until we saw each other again. A permanent move to my home in the summer of 2012 was the next stage for us as a couple.

CHAPTER 3

THE PERFECT MATCH

PETE'S STORY

A few months into our relationship, during a trip to Wembley, Steph finally realised the extent of my footballing background. The fact that she so clearly hadn't a clue about football or what I had achieved in the game was one of the things I found so appealing and endearing about her. By now, Steph knew I had played football professionally, of course, that much was clear enough. But the extent of my history within the sport was something that she remained oblivious about for some time. She wasn't into football. Her dad was a big Ipswich fan, but I don't think she had ever even had a discussion with him about football.

This all changed when I was invited to Wembley for a big event as a guest of the Football Association. England were playing a friendly against Brazil and I was presenting Steven Gerrard with an award — a memento of his 100th cap playing for England. I wanted Steph to attend with me. We were chauffeur-driven straight into the bowels of the stadium and parked up close to the players tunnel and dressing rooms, an area that the FA don't usually make available very often to anyone other than the players themselves. One of the FA staff came out to show me into the room where the trophy was awaiting the pre-match presentation, pointing out that it might have to be a different kind of presentation as the trophy was rather on the heavy side. I asked her whether, as we were on the spot, I could show Steph the pitch and where the dressing rooms were, and she agreed.

As we strolled down the tunnel, there were some pictures of some of England's best players and of course one massive picture of their most capped player – yours truly! Steph was amazed and quite visibly shocked when she spotted the picture of me. "*That's you!*" she gasped. I think the penny had dropped. Steph realised that I had played football at a vastly different level than she had first imagined. "Yes," I told her, "that is me and I have indeed played at Wembley quite a few times in my career for England." We walked out onto the famous pitch. She'd only been there for five minutes and she was standing on the Wembley turf – yes, in her high heels!

Later, before the match began, I went on the pitch to make the presentation and Steph stayed in the tunnel. She watched as both teams came out on to the pitch, which she thought was amazing. I was delighted and honoured to make the presentation. I have always considered Gerrard to be a model professional, and it is a wonderful achievement to reach 100 caps. There are not many of us in that very small club.

I must say that I didn't have fond memories of the day I reached that incredibly proud moment of reaching 100 caps. In fact, it was not something I wanted to recall at all. I was captain of my country's team on that day as we faced Holland in the European Championships. The Dutch team were at the top of their game and were, in fact, one of the best Dutch teams of all time. With players like Ruud Gullit, Frank Rijkaard, and Marco Van Basten who scored an incredible hat-trick, we lost 3–1 and were eliminated from the tournament. Just to make that game even more unbearable, was the fact that I was forced to wear a horrendous black and green zig-zag goalkeeper's jersey. I was supposed to wear the shirt in our first match against Ireland but, because Ireland play in green, there was a colour clash. So I was spared having to wear it then and ended up wearing it against Holland. Nobody had asked me beforehand what I thought of the new strip, it was just thrown at me, so to speak, and I hated it. In fact, I hated everything about that game. It was the only time I wore that jersey and that was about the one good thing about it!

However, that day was a good day for the captain of England. Gerrard and the England team notched up a morale-boosting win against Brazil; only their fourth victory in 24 matches against the five-times World Cup winners. It was incredible to think they had players like Jack Wilshere and Theo Walcott making an impact on the Brazilian defence, in Roy Hodgson's experimental midfield triangle of Gerrard sitting back while Wilshere and Tom Cleverley were given the licence to roam.

It's incredibly difficult to achieve 100 caps and, don't get me wrong, I am immensely proud of joining that exclusive club of England Centurions. You have to be dedicated, consistent and show quality of performance, as well as being lucky with injuries. I am immensely proud of my record – my 125 caps are something I treasure – no one could be more proud to have played for their country. When I reached 100 caps there had only been Billy Wright, Bobby Moore and Bobby Charlton before me. Billy Wright won 105 caps and was the first to reach a century. Bobby Moore reached 108 caps and was the most successful England player to achieve over 100 caps. Bobby Charlton managed 106 caps and, when he retired in 1970, he was the most capped England player. No one thought his record could ever be beaten.

The modern game is now full of internationals against nations and competitions that hadn't even existed in my time, such as the new Nations League, so there are many more opportunities to be capped. There was also a time when England managers handed out caps to a profusion of substitute players, so a player would earn a cap without playing the full 90 minutes or at least the majority of the game. That game against Brazil at Wembley was Gerrard's 101st cap. It was also Ashley Cole's 100th, which made him the seventh English footballer to reach the milestone, but he had to wait until later to receive his 'Golden Cap'. There were two more to hit the 100-mark – Frank Lampard and Wayne Rooney. Lampard played in three World Cups and was the England team's most prolific penalty taker with nine goals. He made his international debut in 1999, went on to score 29 goals and won 106 caps. Rooney came very close to my record, but eventually fell five caps short at 120. David Beckham reached 115 caps. It's hard to imagine that, if Rooney and Beckham failed to reach 125 caps, whether there is anyone who ever will again. It's a fact that of the few to reach 100 caps, I am the only goalkeeper on the list. It is harder for midfield players and forwards to avoid injuries which can cut a career short. Steven Gerrard ended up winning 114 caps but had already had persistent back problems early in his career. Without injury, perhaps Steven could have gone on and represented his country a record number of times.

If anyone was to break my record of 125 caps then I would be the first to congratulate them. Anyone who did manage that would have to love the game, be totally dedicated, determined and hard working. But my 125 caps is not the only record I am proud of. The 1,390 competitive games in my career is the most anyone has managed in world football. I also had it confirmed, whilst researching for this book, that I also hold the all-time record for the most World Cup appearances in world football. My England debut was a match against East Germany in November 1970, but I didn't get round to actually playing my first international tournament until the European Championships in Italy in 1980. I went on to make seventeen appearances at World Cup finals, kept ten clean sheets and captained England to a fourth-place finish at Italia '90 at the age of 40 and that is a world record! Of my 125 appearances for England, 66 resulted in victories. So, not a bad record over my 20-year career playing for my country.

But to be honest, none of that was on my mind as I stood in Wembley that day. I was more interested in ensuring that Steph was being looked after and that she was having a wonderful time. She had been sat next to Sir Bobby Charlton and his wife at the pre-match meal, while I was next to the President of Brazil and his wife. Chatting to the President, the conversation came round to the infamous "Hand of God" incident. It was inevitable, as just about everyone I meet asks me about Diego Maradona's goal in the World Cup in Mexico. It was gratifying to hear the president's thoughts on it. Football is very important for the Brazilian ethos. They believe that it truly is the beautiful game – a game of sportsmanship, heroics, goals and glory… Not a game for cheats. He was horrified that Diego had cheated, and even more horrified that he got away with it. I told him I was still waiting for an apology.

For Steph and me, the next big match would be our wedding. We both wanted the same thing – a white wedding. But we were both set to go through a lot of heartache before we got to that point.

STEPH'S STORY

About six months after we first met, Pete invited me as his guest to an England match at Wembley. He had been invited by the FA to present Steven Gerrard with his 100th cap for England who were playing against Brazil.

I got dressed up and was really looking forward to the event. We had a chauffeur pick us up. When we got there Pete was met by a lady working for the FA who wanted to run through how the presentation would take place before the match started. We were led out on to the famous pitch. I couldn't believe it – I had gone from having no knowledge about football to being shown the dressing rooms of the England team. And now, I was actually being taken out on the pitch at one of the most famous stadiums in the world and the home to English football – in my high heels!

As we were walking down the tunnel you couldn't miss that it was lined with huge images of famous England players. Suddenly, I saw a massive picture of Pete. I was taken aback for a moment and said, "Oh wow, *that's you.*" Pete just laughed and replied, "Yes, I have played here a bit." Typical Pete, so modest.

At the pre-match meal, I was seated next to Sir Bobby Charlton and his wife and they were absolutely lovely, so friendly and kind to me. He asked me what I predicted would happen in the game – something I suppose any ex-player would ask. Obviously, I was distraught as I knew nothing about football so I just thought that I would be honest with him. I told him I had no idea what to expect at the match and that when I first met Pete I thought he was a musician. Bobby found that so amusing that he laughed out loud. "So, please don't ask me about the game, Sir Bobby, because I know nothing about football," I pleaded. "Oh, how refreshing," he said. "What would you like to talk about?" We went on to chat in depth about the NHS which he found fascinating and then about their grandchildren. He and his wife were so easy to talk to and genuinely interested in what I had to say about my career and Pete loved that. Some men might have felt embarrassed that their partner was talking to an England legend and chatting on about the NHS but Pete's not like that. He loves the fact that I am natural and that I can talk to anyone and basically be myself.

When Pete went on to the pitch to make the presentation I was able to stay in the tunnel and watch both teams go out on to the pitch. Seeing the England squad lined up was amazing and I knew it would be every football fan's dream.

It was revealing to see how much respect everyone around had for Pete. It was obvious to me that he was a true footballing hero, but I also admired the fact that he remained so unpretentious and down to earth.

Being guests of the FA, we were seated in the Royal Box which was amazing for me. Walking out and being seated in the front row with 90,000 supporters in the stadium was something very special but, I have to admit, frightening for me. In the Royal Box I was seated next to a really nice man and we started chatting. I asked him if he was a well-known ex-footballer. He laughed at me in a friendly way and replied, "I wish!" It turned out he was David Gill, the Chief Executive of Manchester United. He was so friendly and nice to me and I think this put me at ease. Pete says that I say the funniest things sometimes – he calls them my Bridget Jones moments – and this was a typical one and the game hadn't even started!

During the match Pete kept whispering in my ear about what was happening during the game. I didn't even know which end England were trying to score at! After about ten minutes of watching the action I said to Pete and David that I thought that England's number eight, Jack Wilshere, was really good. Later on, an announcement came over the tannoy that Jack Wilshere had been named Man of the Match. "I said he was good, didn't I?" I reminded David. He laughed and replied, "Yes, I know, Steph, you did. And you were right."

Pete just let me be myself, he didn't tell me how important anyone was or how I was expected to behave, he just wanted me to enjoy myself. It showed the level of trust we had between us. He wanted me to have a good time and knew I wasn't there for the fame game. I had no idea just how famous Pete was until that day and he always says that was one of the reasons he knew we would be together. Despite his world of football being so remote from what I knew, we seemed to work so well together. People really wanted to engage with us as a couple.

At the end of the match, we met Steven Gerrard in the lift. It was his big day and he was the star of the show but he was more interested in meeting Pete and was so respectful towards him. This was the first time that I recognised Pete's stature in football. Working 40–50 hours a week and singing on stage was my world but suddenly I was invited into Pete's world and I got a taste of how successful and admired he was. I came away quite overwhelmed. From then on, my bubble changed forever. In this bizarre new life, some days I found myself sitting in a plush, red leather seat in the Royal Box at Wembley watching England's footballing elite and then the following morning I would be back in my black plastic NHS office chair. I had to get my head around it. I came to see Pete's world like being on stage – the point where I walk out and prepare to perform and sing and then it's back to the normality of home life. And I guess it is that attitude that equipped me to cope with his world. From that match onwards my life changed. And it was never to be the same again.

CHAPTER 4

SIGNS AND SUSPICIONS

STEPH'S STORY

I remember one particular time that I had a very funny betting experience. It was my one and only gambling experience at the horse races. I come from a large, close family and from a very young age I remember that we would have big fun days out. As I grew older we would sometimes have a day at Newmarket racecourse as we didn't live too far from it. It's a beautiful course with a wealth of history and it's known to many as the headquarters of British racing. On the handful of times we went, we would always head for the members' enclosure, close to the pre-race parade ring, the winning post and with access to the grandstand and the paddock enclosure. My sister, Claire, and I would always thoroughly look forward to these occasions and would get very dressed up for them. We always enjoyed watching the horses being paraded around the pre-parade ring – it was such a treat. We'd sit there trying to pick the winner.

On this particular occasion we decided that we were going to bet on a horse in every race that day. We worked out that we could each afford £5 per race and we were convinced we would make a great return. Usually in the members' enclosure there are Totes to place your bets with but, for a giggle, we decided to run down and sneak through the barriers to the bookies that stand by the track in the garden enclosure. The first bookie was a real character – a trench-coated cockney – and we decided to place our bets on the first race with him. Looking completely out of place in our smart attire and high heels we quickly ran like mad back to the members' area to wait at the winning post and watch the race, only to see our horse lose.

After that, we again scrambled through the crowds back down to the same bookie to place our bet on the next race and again ran back to the winning post. This activity continued for every race – same bookie, same outcome. We were determined to win our money back from the cockney.

On the very last race we went down to the bookie to place our final bet and were thrilled when he said, "No, girls, you can have this one on me – free." Claire and I assured each other that Lady Luck was now on our side. But in picking winners, we were hopeless. We lost that race too and we were exhausted. We had no clue what we were doing, but it really made us laugh. We had had a wonderful fun day out and to this day we still end up in hysterics with our mum remembering that experience. How on earth we could have lost on *every single* race at the meeting?

One a serious note, what I learned from that day is that there was no such thing as a free bet. My experience of gambling was losing not winning. The cockney set the scene for me and I'm sure it was the same for my sister. If you want to lose money, place a bet.

That was my limited experience with betting, but my experience of addiction was more extensive and came from the time I worked in the Special Care Baby Unit in the hospital. Here, I learned a lot about how it affected whole families. In the unit we were caring for mothers with addictions and whose newborn babies had to be weaned off drugs such as heroin and alcohol that, sadly, their mothers had been so hooked on they couldn't do without, even throughout their pregnancies. The children are born addicts and it's devastating to see. I'd often spend time talking to the mothers. It was heartbreaking as, for both the mum and the baby, the withdrawal process was long and so difficult. Babies need to be slowly weaned off and they go through terrible withdrawal symptoms. Managing the administration in that department meant that I was surrounded by addiction issues and I wasn't afraid to look at that dark place in life. Over the years, I worked my way up the ladder and began to do more work dealing with consultants and GPs so my view on life became quite clinical. I would think nothing of working sixteen-hour days. I thrived in my career and I worked with some wonderful, dedicated and hardworking individuals. But during my time in the Special Baby Care Unit, it never occurred to me to link gambling addiction with substance addictions. Little did I know how that particular addiction could become such a horrible, horrendous experience in anyone's life let alone my own. Yes, gambling doesn't tend to affect newborn babies but sadly it does touch the lives of thousands of older children and young people.

At the time, I was living in a Victorian town house on the outskirts of Colchester, very close to restaurants, cafes and boutiques. The house was open plan with an open beamed staircase that spiralled into the lounge area. The property was also within easy walking distance of Colchester town centre and only a 20-minute drive to the surrounding coastal areas. Pete loved the area as people were far more discreet in recognising him than he had been used to, it was a very cosmopolitan part of the town. Pete and I were together and life was idyllic. We were madly in love and both working professionally. We had a great social life together – it was perfect – and we had started living together in our blissfully happy bubble.

But it wasn't long before the first tiny warning signs of his problem started to appear. There was a time, prior to us moving in together, that I remember getting a call from Pete at 2 a.m. and he sounded very down – in an extremely low mood. I heard an emptiness in his voice. He seemed so down and depressed. I thought it was because he was feeling lonely and missed me, but I later realised it was likely because he had experienced a day and night of bad losses. I was incredibly sad for him. I ended the telephone call by saying to Pete; "I promise you'll never be lonely again and I will always be there for you." I could tell he was in a very dark place.

I used to do everything I could to make Pete feel special, because he is. I wanted him to know that I would be by his side to support and protect him. Since the time we'd first met he had always looked after me, so I wanted to do the same for him. The first birthday of his that we celebrated as a couple, I took him out to lunch and wanted to spoil him. I picked a lovely restaurant and had organised balloons for the table, ready for when we arrived. I could tell he was really pleased. During the meal he visited the toilet and, whilst he was gone, I put his present on the table. I'd had it beautifully gift wrapped with a bow and ribbons. And inside the box was an Armani watch. When he returned he opened his gift and he literally started to well up with tears. I chose a watch because I had noticed that he had a very ordinary one and deserved something a bit more stylish. It was a beautiful watch and I thought it was perfect for him and one that he could wear for work. He was so choked up that it surprised me, but it was lovely to see his reaction. Most people would have simply said: "Oh this is lovely, thank you" but Pete was visibly taken aback and very emotional. He later revealed to me that it was the first time he had been emotional over his birthday. He'd had this reputation as a macho man, but he melted when he realised that someone cared for him. He was definitely overwhelmed on that day.

I was brought up in a family where birthdays and Christmas are big celebrations, filled with love and gifts – so, to me, this was a normal thing to do for someone you love. I realised that this gift was so special for Pete because it showed just how much I loved him. It wasn't just the watch that he loved but the gesture behind it. He really appreciated it. For a moment, I questioned in my mind if no one had really cared for him before.

There was so much Pete had missed out on during his life. In his playing days, days like Christmas and Bank Holidays were filled with training and matches. For Pete, his life had been his career and gambling – nothing in between – but now it was different. I guess I wanted to show him that life could be special and that I loved him.

After a couple of months of living together, I started to notice a strangeness to Pete's behaviour. He would often go out of the room to be on his phone and it obviously crossed my mind that maybe he was seeing another woman. It naturally made me suspicious. If he was watching TV he would often quickly change the channel whenever I appeared in the room. The remote control was never far from his hands. If it wasn't another woman then why was his behaviour so edgy and shifty? I became paranoid and convinced that something was going on. I had to get to the bottom of it so, one day, I asked if I could borrow his phone as mine wasn't charged up. I quickly sifted through his call history and there was one number that cropped up time and time again. I wrote it down. Later, I nervously rang it. It was a gambling company. It was at that moment that it all fell into place. Pete was gambling. I knew that now. But it would still take a while for me to uncover the staggering extent of his gambling addiction. For now, I was just confused as to why he would hide it from me.

I decided to attempt approaching the subject of gambling with Pete. We were out at a Chinese restaurant for lunch. I had noticed, on previous occasions, that if we went out for lunch he would become jittery and want to get home. I decided to be frank, so I said to him: "Pete, I don't know anything about football, but I've been to Newmarket races and I certainly know who Henry Cecil is. Do you like betting on the horses?" He then admitted to me that he liked a little flutter on the horses. I said: "That's great but you don't have to sneak around and watch the horse racing behind my back. You can do it in front of me." He seemed really relieved that day and he relaxed completely. For once, he didn't rush our lunch. I thought the problem was solved and he obviously thought, 'Great, no more ducking and diving and hiding this from Steph.' I just wanted him to be himself, and not feel like he had to lead a double life. Problem solved. Or so I thought…

Pete wasn't hiding his gambling from me now and it didn't take long for me to see the extent of it. From that point onwards, I was able to start piecing things together and I began to suspect it was an addiction. All of a sudden, his strange, secretive behaviour made sense. I decided to become an 'investigator' and ascertain exactly how bad Pete's gambling was. The signs were all there – if he wasn't working then his time and attention centred around horse racing. I became very uneasy about it all. I did wonder if maybe I could be overthinking things. Was I reading too much into it all? However, my gut feelings kept shouting at me – "ADDICTION" – so, for my own sanity, I had to uncover the truth.

CHAPTER 5

THE GAMBLER

PETE'S STORY

From a very young age, probably about eight or nine years old, football was my life. All I wanted to be was a professional player and my parents supported me 100 per cent, in any way they could because we weren't a rich family. My dad, Les, ran a grocery shop with my mum, May, and they worked really hard. They were both born and bred in Leicester, and were very loving and supportive parents and totally grounded individuals.

My fondest memories of my childhood are of our family holidays. Mum and Dad bought a good-sized static caravan just after the mid-1950s. It was situated at a holiday caravan park right on the beachfront in Trusthorpe, a small coastal village just two miles from Mablethorpe, East Lincolnshire. The location was ideal as it was only two and a half hours from our Leicester home. The campsite was a lovely small site. Just a few hundred yards up a slope was the sea and the beach. Not only did we have summer holidays there, but sometimes Dad would shut up the shop on a late Saturday afternoon and we would be there for teatime, returning back late on the Sunday night. Heading to the caravan was always so exciting for me and I fondly remember Mum and Dad would be just as excited. It was their getaway place from all the hard work they did in a built-up city. It became our happy haven.

The excitement would begin when we started packing the car. And there was one thing I'd never forget to take with me – my precious football. We had the holiday home from when I was about eight years old up until my mid-teens and I never once forgot the football. Every single Christmas of my childhood, all I ever wanted was a new football, a new football kit and football annuals. I can still recall the strong smell of leather of my new football and my football boots on Christmas Day. Football was my Christmas wish from the age of seven onwards.

Our holiday breaks would be filled with fun times; crabbing with Dad, swimming in the sea as a family with my brother who is five years younger than me, but mainly the memories are of being goalie on the beach. Me and my dad used to mount the sand up into two sandcastles that would act as goalposts and I'd get Dad to shoot and make crosses at me – even at that age the love of the game was there. Other children and their dads visiting the beach would always join in. Even at just nine years old I didn't want to let a goal in. My dad was amazed so see grown men trying their best to get the ball past me. The other dads would sometimes comment to my dad "Christ, he's good" and Dad would smile and nod. Dad never pushed or put pressure on me – he was my silent supporter. He was always gently encouraging and that's why I grew up to believe that parents should never pressurise their children in sport. Back at home, I was desperate to get into the Leicester school under-11s area team, which I did at the age of ten.

As well as great times on the beach we used to have long walks to the funfair in Mablethorpe. We'd often sit in pub gardens, my brother and I drinking pop. Then we'd pick up a fish and chip takeaway on the way home. The memory that I spoke of in the introduction to this book comes from one of these stays at our caravan holiday home. Very occasionally Dad used to like to have a flutter on the horses and on holiday he would pop out to the bookie in Mablethorpe and place his bets while Mum would take me and my brother to the arcade. Dad had apparently been given some tips on the horses running that week. On the last day of our holiday, Dad put a bet of £10 each way on a horse which was 12 to 1. Dad had seemed to be on a lucky streak all week – he already had five horses come in first. So he decided to make a big bet on the last race. In those days £10 was a lot of money. I clearly remember the sight of my dad running like hell towards us with a huge grin on his face, shaking his hands in the air. He had won again. We were all so excited – totally elated – that Dad had won so much money. We all went to the pub, sat in the garden and celebrated. I remember Dad treating us and Mum with his winnings. That holiday really stuck out for me.

There was another earlier time that my dad won that stuck in my memory. It was a day out at Windsor races. I must have been about six or seven years old and I remember Dad holding my hand as we ran to the winning post. Because there were so many people and I was so small I couldn't see anything but suddenly I felt the thud of galloping horses on the ground and a cry out as Dad said his horse had won. He had put a £2 bet on a 25 to 1 horse. Again, there was great excitement for me and my dad at the win. It's strange though that, when I reflect back, despite Dad not being an addict I had a strong sense that Mum didn't like him gambling.

They say people get into gambling by either having or seeing someone get a big win. Maybe these were the moments that triggered my interest in gambling. Unfortunately, I didn't learn the lesson to keep my cash safe. The one thing I was never taught was the value of money and the dangers of gambling but I don't blame Mum and Dad because it was in my DNA anyway. And attitudes were different towards gambling and bookmakers back then. People weren't fully aware of the risks and the dangers.

In the '80s and '90s when my gambling really accelerated I would have accounts with the three big bookmakers – Ladbrokes, William Hill and Coral. Each account had a credit limit put on them of £9,000 to £10,000 and when I reached that limit my betting had to stop until I had paid that off. I would have summaries of my accounts sent to me every two weeks when I was supposed to pay them. Sometimes I needed extra time to raise the money to do that. The limits didn't stop me having big losses but at least I had to settle up before I could bet again. During those pre-internet days, I would be on a landline phone to place my bets and would listen to the racing commentary on the radio. The only TV coverage of the horse racing was on the BBC. Sometimes, if all my accounts were at their limits, I would then bet in cash at a bookmaker. It was never good to be seen in a bookmakers shop as people talk so I preferred to bet privately using the phone. Even then, I was very secretive about my gambling.

When my career in football came to an end, it was the age of the internet and the new online exchange betting started which revolutionised the gambling world. Back then I was not someone that had much interest in the internet, but I took a look. The changes were really exciting for a committed gambler like myself, with so many different things to bet on. I could now bet on *every* sport around the world, 24 hours a day. It was totally different. You weren't limited to betting only on a win but also for a horse to lose. This opened up for some people to cheat – that is conspiring to stop a horse from winning and profiting from the loss. I started using this new betting exchange in 2006. After a few years of mostly low-key betting the old way, I was suddenly hooked again. I could sit with the computer and bet as much as I wanted. At the time I was working in a few different areas – as an after-dinner and a motivational speaker – but I still had lots of time to gamble. And I started to dedicate even more hours to it – I wanted to be professional at my horse betting and started studying the form even more.

Of course, all the effort I put in was in vain as I still lost money regularly and losses came more easily on the exchanges. You could transfer money in and out of accounts in a flash so now there were no limits to my losses. The exchange betting companies keep your account details on record for you to check so I knew the exact extent of my losses. That never stopped me gambling more though.

When it came to my career in football, I was totally dedicated and wouldn't let anything get in the way. I would give the game 100 per cent both mentally and physically. The best goalkeepers are the ones who make the fewest mistakes, and I feel that I played so well and had such an exceptional career because I was willing to give everything I had to achieve that. Perhaps I am unique in that respect. I trained exceptionally hard, and often stayed behind for extra training. If I conceded a goal, I would analyse it over and over again to learn from my mistake and constantly improve my game.

From the '60s to the '90s, there were no goalkeeping coaches. I would train myself with different technique methods and training routines – more than just a bit of shooting and crossing that keepers did in those days.

Football was always number one in my life and I worked very hard to be successful. I never rushed away from training to watch a race I had a bet on. I never sacrificed training and preparation for a game for my gambling. I was always focused. You might be able to coast through a game in some positions but not as a goalkeeper. Make one mistake as keeper and it could cost your team the match. It is often said that a team with a very good goalkeeper is worth fifteen points a season.

So, football came first.

But I also had my secret world. I would place a bet in the morning and wait until I could see a re-run of the race later in the day. I was quite disciplined in that way – it was part of my personality. When I was on a break from playing, I would sit by the phone and have a bet. If there was night racing in the summer, I'd bet on that. Whenever I went on holiday I would always order the English newspapers so I could study the form and keep up to date on the results for when I got home. I never had a bet on holiday as I wanted a complete rest – again I saw this as part of my discipline.

In both these worlds I thought of myself as a perfectionist – a perfectionist in whatever I did. But, while I had control over my training and the games, I had no control over the gambling. I had a great life in football. I achieved everything I wanted to, won everything apart from the FA Cup – although I was on a team that reached the final in 1969. But, in total contrast, off the pitch my life was gradually disintegrating.

I could keep my betting and my football career separate but the betting meant all my other business activities ended in tears. My gambling had a bad knock-on effect on everything else I set up in my business life outside of football. On the field, nothing affected my game, I was far too focused to allow that to happen. But, behind the scenes away from the game, I was betting all the time and that became a major drain on my finances.

At that time I blamed everything except myself and my gambling habits, which is a typical response from gamblers who are no longer in control of their addiction. Instead, I tried to lay the blame on the falling housing market, but the truth is that while there was a dip in the housing market that contributed to my downfall, it was the gambling that ensured I wasn't able to prop it up. I just didn't have the resources to do so.

It became a different world out there for the gambling industry with the internet – more advertising, a growing number of internet betting companies and more temptation. Gambling became even more hidden and secretive. There were times of high jubilation and you would want to tell the world that you were a winner, but invariably those times were outnumbered by the losses. And, if you were a loser, you remained secretive about that. You would think that these companies would have a duty of care to their clients, would alert them when they suspect they are betting too much and, more to the point, losing more than they could afford. But no. No way. On the contrary, if they detect regular winners on their platforms, bookmakers will reduce their stakes or close down their accounts entirely.

The majority of my gambling was on horse racing although I once trained greyhounds and even bred a couple, during my days at Leicester City. Back then, my routine was to pop into the bookies for the odd bet now and again. But my passion was for horse racing. I loved going to the races and ended up owning and racing my own horses – around half a dozen of them.

I've never been interested in roulette. For me that's just about guessing on red or black so there isn't much skill in it, and I've never really taken to the casino atmosphere. I tried it once in a very posh restaurant and casino in Nottingham. The meal was lovely, but I didn't take to the roulette. In contrast, I think there is a skill to the horses – you study the form, think about the going and the factors that might help your bet come in. Similarly, with card games which some teammates enjoyed on England trips in the early '70s there was a skill to the game. There used to be something called a Brag school which involved Joe Royle, Kevin Keegan, Malcolm Macdonald, Emlyn Hughes, Mick Channon and Frank Worthington. In those days we stayed overnight before returning to our clubs the next day after a match. The Brag school card games usually went on into the early hours of the morning and those who lost had to carry their losses over to the away fixture. Later on in my England career there were other card playing groups but, as far as I know, nothing that ended with big losses. Poker is a game I have never played but I see there is a lot of skill involved which is why so many professional players make a good living from it. I would have the odd bet when away playing with England, but I always kept it a small amount as nothing interfered with my preparations for the game.

Racing was something I told myself was a hobby, a form of relaxation but I also thought of myself as a sort of 'professional' gambler because

I took the time to study the form and come to an educated decision on where I would place my money. After I retired from football, my agent even booked me to open a betting shop. Yep, you couldn't make it up, could you? But people knew I liked a bet. To be fair, no one knew to what extent my gambling was becoming a problem, so I am not blaming anyone for the fact that I was hired to open the Coral high street branch. I tended to use the phone to place bets so, when I went into this betting shop, it was quite an eye-opener. I did my 'meet and greet'. I didn't have a bet, of course, as I was working, so I could detach myself from the gambling for that moment. But I did notice there were four FOBT (Fixed Odds Betting Terminals) in the shop, all of them fully occupied with punters. The machines enable fast pace gambling with free spins — a lot like the roulette wheels that never appealed to me. They have since been described as the "crack cocaine" of gambling. At that time the limit was £100 a spin. The punters were steadily pumping money into these machines. Thankfully new legislation introduced in 2018 has reduced the stake on these machines to £2.

Perhaps the biggest win I had in my playing career was when I placed a £500 bet and won £33,000. I recall another time that had a £1,000 bet on a treble and won £40,000 with an independent bookie. Naturally he wasn't happy, but I managed to put the smile back on his face because, within a few weeks I gave it all back to him. Those kinds of wins were few and far between. And every single penny I won went back to the bookies as I placed more and more bets chasing that winning feeling. It's for the wins, those moments, those amazing highs, that's the reason you gamble. Unfortunately, there are far more crashing lows.

At one time, during the '90s, I found myself £60,000 up with my William Hill account whilst I was having an exceptionally good run. Although they sent a statement confirming my account was in credit, they declined to pay me on time. Their reason? Well, they pointed out the times I had been slow to pay when my account was in deficit. As it was it didn't matter because, over a short period of time, I lost that amount and gave them that much back again and more. That £60k quickly disappeared from a credit to a debt again. In fact, in one of my wild days in the '90s, I lost £20,000 in just one day.

For me, not only was there an adrenalin rush of excitement when I won, but also when I lost, because there was the thrill of thinking I would then find a winner to recoup the losses. One thing was certain, win or lose, I would have another bet. The very nature of a gambler means that even winning isn't enough, you go back for more until you have blown your winnings and start a losing streak. You're always compelled to keep going and feeding the money back into bets. Naturally money feeds the habit. If you have £10 spare, you will bet £10, if you have £100 burning a hole in your pocket you will bet the £100. And so on, to the point that if you happened to have £1 million spare, then you will bet that without blinking. It is what it says on the tin – you are a gambler: committed and addicted.

I earned good money at the top of my game and was one of the highest paid footballers of my time, but I spent it as soon as it came in. Don't get me wrong, I still lived a nice lifestyle with houses, holidays and horses but, as my gambling habit took a hold on my life, the money was disappearing as quickly as I was earning it. And that was something I kept very secret, I was silent about it, all the time thinking that I would soon enough hit the jackpot and recoup those heavy losses. When those jackpots popped up from time to time, they were all I needed to kid myself that wins might happen again and again. They don't.

In sport, where professionals should be setting an example, I believe gambling is now as rife as it was in my time in the '70s, '80s and '90s, maybe even worse. Gamblers who are out of control become secretive and silent. Sometimes problems become public when a celebrated figure is revealed to have made a very large loss. There have been many well-known people who have been reported as or eventually confessed to being heavy gamblers. But for all those who come clean, there are literally thousands who keep it all quiet. Just like those who take drugs or drink to excess, they keep it all a secret for as long as they can, so no one really knows the full extent of the problem until it's too late. But, of course, wealthy people can afford it. Or they *think* they can, until they find out far too late that they can't. As I've said, money fuels gambling.

Gambling is rife in sports such as football. In football you can earn a lot of money and also have a lot of spare time on your hands after training and between matches which can so often turn into boredom. You find yourself looking for something to occupy you when you are tired after games and training. When I was playing football, I chose not to walk around a golf course or a similar pastime, so I convinced myself that gambling was a hobby – a form of relaxation for my spare time. After games that physically push you to extremes and then all the training, you need periods of rest, and something to fill those quiet periods. Internet gambling especially is an easy and tempting option. Gambling can also be an extension of the high you get playing your sport. Sportsmen who are highly competitive want to keep that adrenalin running, they want to keep on a high and gambling fills that need.

The problems for all people who find themselves addicted to gambling – not just millionaire footballers – can escalate rapidly. Gambling addicts can face deep and terrible depressions. There are increasing cases of addicts resorting to crime or fraud to keep themselves afloat financially or even resorting to suicide in extreme circumstances. Gambling is an illness – and we already have an epidemic on our hands. This needs to be faced head on.

I should know, because I now accept how much I suffered with acute depression over my gambling and my losses. I acknowledge now how tough it was to keep such a dark secret to myself. I had an illness but didn't know it. I felt guilt, but I also felt on a high when I was gambling. I couldn't stop because I told myself I couldn't afford to stop. Most people have become aware of the effects of alcohol and drugs, but not so much with gambling, although there are many similarities. Gambling – like substance abuse – is very dangerous for mental and physical health. I was suffering deep down but always kept a brave face and I think this is true of a lot of gambling addicts. Behind that façade, gambling was overtaking my life. It will take over the life of any gambler who is betting out of control. You structure your entire day around your betting habit from the minute you wake up – even if that entire day entails just one bet. Your whole mindset from the moment you wake up to the moment you go to sleep. You feel overpowered by the need to bet to the point where it becomes so emotional that you feel fatigued by the sheer effort of placing the bets. It becomes so time-consuming that you have little time, if any, for much else in life.

Gambling became a much larger force in my life when I retired from football. Playing football detached me from the gambling world. With football, even if my team lost a game I would never get down about it. I was a true professional and always strived to make the very best possible performance in my next game. Also, when you are a professional footballer the physical exercises are the best possible antidepressant you can give yourself. When I retired, I had no football and the routine it involved to distract me at the very time when slick and easy betting via the internet opened another door for my gambling.

With sports in America and Australia continuing through the night, it meant that if you didn't have a great day betting here in the UK, there was always the other side of the world to try to make up for your losses. By the time you feel ready to sleep, you are exhausted with all the effort, leaving you tired and emotional. It is not healthy for your mind or body. Fortunately, I never felt suicidal, but I realise now I did suffer from depression at that time. My emotions were like a yo-yo – I would go from the high of a win to the low mood of subsequent losses. I would go into myself becoming almost reclusive. On nights where I had had big losses it seriously affected my sleep, so I suffered a lot of restless nights over the years that I gambled. There were times during my addiction that I would literally be physically sick in the bathroom first thing in the morning at the thought of what I had lost the day or the night before.

Deep down I felt I had a void in my life that needed filling and, without the football, I guess that feeling was exposed so the dark place was able to engulf me more. I'm quite a strong personality – I showed that throughout my football career – so I convinced myself I could handle the emotions and the pressures in my life brought about by my gambling losses. As a goalkeeper, if you made errors and had to live with them, overcome them, put them to the back of your mind and get on with it.

Being a goalkeeper is a lonely life, a lot of responsibility rests on your shoulders alone. I thought I was built to handle the ups and downs of football and goalkeeping, so I thought I could handle the ups and downs that came with gambling. Only now I realise that I couldn't.

When football ceased to be the main force in my life, gambling took centre stage and led to depression. With depression I began to drink more than I used to – more than I should have done. I felt lethargic – thinking all day and every day about gambling was exhausting. It was my waking thought and my last thought at night. Gambling and the hold it can get on an addict can end relationships, ruin careers and destroy lives.

It was only when I met Steph that I finally recognised the void I had been trying to fill. I finally saw that it could be filled by something other than gambling. With her by my side, I felt so much happier in my life. Looking back, this was the beginning of my battle to end my addiction. But it would not be an easy fight.

CHAPTER 6

LIVING WITH THE ADDICT

STEPH'S STORY

Pete's obsession with betting was confined to horses and he had a background in the sport. I've since learned that many footballers and ex-players are gambling addicts. It appears to be a world that they are attracted to and, with so much spare time on their hands and money to play with, they become easy prey for the gambling companies and bookmakers to pull in.

By then I knew that Pete was using his mobile phone to bet on horse racing, but I started to notice that he was using a laptop while watching the racing on TV. Again, every time I walked into the lounge the laptop would quickly be closed. After a while, it became obvious to me that the laptop was also one of his betting tools. I couldn't understand what the link was, so 'Ms Investigator' needed to start delving into it. Trying to find out the truth about Pete's gambling had become a silent game of cat and mouse. How was I going to get into the laptop? If I asked Pete about it he responded in the usual way – he would block me out and change the subject. I was certain that laptop would be the key to unlocking my gambling concerns over Pete.

Obviously, he had password protected the laptop so there was no way I could log on to it without that. Late one evening, I tiptoed very quietly halfway down the stairs. The lounge is open-plan so I could see into it. Bingo! There was Pete watching a race on the TV with his laptop open, unaware that I was hiding on the stairs. I could see the screen and digitally it was the same as the ones I'd seen at Newmarket races – a gambling Tote. So, he didn't need to rely on his phone to bet. He had obviously been using his phone at the start of our relationship so that he could discreetly pop outside and listen to the races.

On the laptop he quite clearly had direct access to online betting. I looked at the TV and he was watching a live horse race in Australia. Suddenly, I realised there was a whole new world of betting that I had not known about. A world that was open for Pete to gamble on races anywhere in the world – America, Australia, literally any horse race – and anytime.

I tiptoed back to bed, realising I had been completely naive about the world of gambling. At that time, I didn't have a smartphone or a home computer only a work computer in my office and private use was strictly forbidden in the NHS back then. So, my next mission was to get into the laptop. I needed to have a good look at his betting account.

Luckily, after a while, the laptop started going wrong so I suggested to Pete that we could buy a far better replacement together so that we could both use it. He couldn't really not agree because what reason could he give for not wanting to share a laptop? Begrudgingly, he did. So, our new laptop was set up and, in my ignorance, I thought "Great, I'm going to be about to see his betting details." How wrong I was. The betting icon was set up on the homepage, but it was heavily password protected. Finding that password would have to be my next mission.

Unknown to me at the time, cracking the password would be an impossible mission. I must admit I did try several times to guess it which led to it being locked. After all my hard work I still couldn't get into the betting account and I was still no closer to knowing the extent of Pete's problems or his financial status, but I wasn't going to quit.

All the signs that Pete was a gambling addict were there and I would tell any loved one in my position to look out for those signs. At first glimpse, a gambler is not as easy to spot as a smoker or drinker or drug user. You can smell smoke on someone. You can smell alcohol on someone's breath or spot that they are drunk by their body movements or hear it in their speech. It's often the same with drugs. But a vulnerable gambler is harder to identify by their physical appearance. A gambler is quite capable of looking you in the eye and telling you nothing is wrong. They're adept at keeping their secrets in the dark. They are like swans; on the surface everything seems calm but underneath they are paddling like mad to try to keep afloat.

If you are worried about a partner having a gambling problem there are signs you can identify. Look out for them being secretive about their phone or computer. Like me, many of these signs might make you wonder if your partner is cheating on you, so you will feel suspicious. They will guard their phone, often not allowing you to see or use it. If you question them about money they will react defensively, often shutting the conversation down immediately. They also divert from the subject and change the direction of conversations – something they master the art of doing. They are not as open and casual as most people would be with each other in a relationship. They tend to become loners and can have poor relationships with friends. You may even hear that they've fallen out with people and that's often because they have borrowed money and not repaid it. Mood swings are another sign – one minute they are high and the next they are low and introverted. If they have a winning run they are so happy that they become the life and soul of the party. They might suggest going out and having a drink or an expensive meal. There's presents and treats. They want to have a good time because they want to celebrate but they can't tell you why. If they've lost big, their mood will suddenly switch and their behaviour will become irrational and irritable. They can be very moody. They will be secretive about their finances and will tell lies, mainly about where the money has gone. And they will be able to find good excuses to ask for money.

Just after the England game at Wembley, Pete brought his parents, May and Les, down to Essex for a visit to meet me. We arranged a few days with them at a hotel on the coast. Those few days were truly wonderful, Pete's parents were such a warm, lovely couple with hearts of gold. I bonded with them immediately. His mum commented several times how pleased she was to see Pete so happy and in love. On the second day Pete took his mum into a shop so I sat on a bench with his dad, looking out at the sea. His dad said to me, "You know Pete has had gambling problems?" I replied, "Yes, I do." His eyes filled with tears as he told me how, over the years, he had seen Pete suffer with it but couldn't find a way to help him. Pete would shut the conversation down. I looked at Les and said, "I will always look after him. I'll never hurt him, and I promise you I'll get him to quit." Les held my hand and responded, "That's music to my ears and I do believe you will."

From then on, I knew I had to fulfil my promise to Les. I was determined. It hit me that Pete had been an addict for all his adult life. I felt heartbroken for him. I realised Pete did have people in his world who loved and cared about him but, due to the addiction, he had clearly built a fortress around himself with a firmly locked door.

A year after we met, Pete proposed. We were going out for Sunday lunch and I noticed he was a little bit quiet and slightly nervous. He suggested we have a couple of drinks before lunch at a wine bar. I thought he drank his first pint of ale rather quickly while I had barely started on my glass of prosecco. As we walked to the restaurant, we passed Colchester Town Hall which is a beautiful building. Pete walked up and stood on the steps of the hall, pulling me gently with him and then, suddenly, he went down on one knee. There, in the middle of the street, in the middle of the daytime, Pete said, "Will you marry me?" I was so shocked as it came out of nowhere but immediately I answered, "Yes, of course." Pete was so relieved. He then sheepishly admitted that he didn't have a ring as he wanted me to choose one myself.

We had lunch at Mussi's, a lovely Italian restaurant. We were both ecstatic and had a nice bottle of wine to celebrate. It was so romantic. But Pete still made me laugh when he said, "I'm so glad I've got that over and done with." We went shopping for the ring a few days later. It was so thoughtful of him to let me choose the one I liked. I picked a beautiful cushion diamond solitaire and we put it on in the shop then and there.

I was on cloud nine – so, so happy – but, in my gut, I couldn't get rid of this terrible feeling that Pete was suffering an addiction and it felt like a massive problem hanging over us. I knew then that this would be a very long engagement as there was no way I was getting married while the addiction was in our lives. His financial situation as a gambler could seriously affect my own financial stability and that scared me. I understood that, the minute we were husband and wife, I would be liable for any debts Pete had run up.

I had had a very well-balanced upbringing. I had been taught the value of money from a young age. I remember a time when I was thirteen years old and all my friends were getting 50p a week pocket money. I asked my dad if I could start to have pocket money. He told me, "I'll think about it." The following day he came home from work and said, "I've sorted out your pocket money, you're going to get a pound a week. I've got you a paper round down at the village newsagents and you start tomorrow." I was ecstatic. Then Dad opened a children's saving account for me and advised me to put 25p a week into my savings. I felt so rich and I learned one of the most valuable lessons in life: that, if I wanted nice things in life, I had to earn them. I had also been taught to be fair, kind, have respect for others and to have my wits about me. Through my career, I had seen for myself what addiction can do to a family and, although I was blissfully happy and in love with Pete, I wouldn't allow myself to be swept away. Of course, I couldn't share my concerns with him.

Nevertheless, our wedding day was something we had both dreamt about. Pete's dream was to take me to Barbados so he said the honeymoon would have to be there. We talked about the wedding day and it became obvious that it was going to cost a lot of money. I used these discussions to remind Pete that when we had everything sorted financially, then we could discuss it properly. I kept telling him that once we had saved enough money we could make all our dreams come true. I was quietly trying to put him under pressure to stop gambling by keep telling him that we would have to wait and save. I wanted to make my vows to God on our special day as much as he did but that wasn't going to happen while there was this cloud over us. I knew, in my heart, that our dreams couldn't become a reality while he was caught up in the web of gambling addiction.

Again, I felt that we were playing a silent game of cat and mouse. I wanted to help Pete, but I also needed to protect myself. I needed to find out what was happening financially for him. I began to recognise when he'd lost and when he'd won. With the joint laptop I thought I would be able to trace his online betting history, but he quickly learnt how to cover his tracks and delete the details. If you want to help a loved one with a gambling addiction you must become an investigator and that's what I became. But you must also prepare yourself for some shocks and heartache.

There is a saying that a gambling addict will "pound for a pound" meaning they will go to any lengths to get hold of money. They are constantly tapping up people to borrow from them. Money is what feeds the addiction and addicts do a fantastic job of finding money to gamble with. They are also highly adept at hiding their sources of money from loved ones. Pete closely guarded his finances from me and kept everything secret. He was leading a double life. For me, life was becoming an emotional roller coaster.

Having decided I needed to protect myself financially, I told Pete that I had got rid of my Barclaycard, but I hadn't. My advice to anyone living with an addict is to never have a joint bank account. I kept mine separate and I kept all my financial details a secret from him. I lied and I told him I didn't have any savings because he could try to tap into that. I told him I would never lend him money.

Pete was always more relaxed and happier at the start of the month, then often looked grey and withdrawn by the end of the month. I knew this flowed from the financial pattern. I saw him watch a race once and he was on the edge of the seat the whole time. He was fixated and his breathing was heavy and laboured. I began to worry about his health. I could clearly see it was an illness and was severely interfering with his well-being. I honestly believe gambling addicts are at an increased risk of strokes and heart attacks and this was something I feared might happen to Pete.

It was at this point that Pete's behaviour started to have an effect on me. I had a very stressful job, and I was living with a man with a now obvious addiction. With the added pressure that this man was famous – I couldn't talk to family or friends about it and I was worried about it coming out in the press if I told anyone other than them. I felt I would be a burden, and that no one would understand. I felt I had nowhere to turn. Also, I wondered if people would be unsympathetic as very few people see gambling addiction as an illness. I couldn't talk to Pete's GP for advice or the bank or the betting company he used because of data protection. I couldn't talk to anyone. I felt embarrassed as there is such a stigma around gambling. I had a sense of shame. This has to change because no one should ever feel like this – alone and unable to find help. I felt that if I told anyone they would judge me and just tell me to leave him and not take on that pressure. But there was no way I was going to leave him to face it on his own – I loved him so much.

I tried to get him to talk about his finances, but every time it was like a door slammed shut and I was totally locked out. Whenever I tried to talk to him about the gambling it was made very clear to me that it was not open to discussion so there was no point in me pursuing it. Pete would always change the subject. He wouldn't even say how much he earned from this job or that job, he would always fudge the details. Secrecy had become a large part of his life and by now that was the norm to me.

I knew he could have a secure and solid future with me, but he was so caught up in the downward spiral of addiction that he couldn't face revealing the enormity of his illness to me or even to himself. During those days, I'd often lay in bed and cry, not just for myself but more for him. I felt so sorry for him. How could this amazing world legend be in this situation? He had achieved so much in his career, but now he was sinking. What a weight he had had to carry around for so many years through those decades. He was so vulnerable, and the addiction was making him ill.

I couldn't see a way to break down the walls Pete had spent 45 years building up around himself and get him to open up. Coming from a clinical world, I knew I would have to deal with this brick by brick. I accepted that it would take time. He was never going to admit to me that he was a chronic gambler and I wondered where it would all end. I loved him and would never have given him an ultimatum – that wasn't the answer. If I'm being completely honest, my deepest fear was the thought that, if I left him, he might take his own life as all he would be left with was himself and the dark world of the addiction. That thought terrified me.

CHAPTER 7

THE IMPACT

PETE'S STORY

I can't tell you how much I have lost over 45 years of a gambling addiction – it must run into the millions. And for a sportsman of my generation – even a footballer at the top end of the country's earners in the sport – it was more than I could afford. On top of the gambling losses there was the loss of a small fortune through my outside businesses. At the height of my playing career, I started what I thought would be a thriving housing portfolio. At its peak, I owned five houses. I also owned a string of racehorses. A downturn in the housing market came at a time when my betting was also getting out of control I found myself unable to support the mortgages on the properties or continue to fund the hugely expensive stable of horses. The drop in value of the houses meant that they landed in negative equity so I couldn't even sell them off to clear the debts. At the time, I told myself I was desperately unlucky, but the reality is that being one of the country's top wage earners at the peak of my playing career, I might have been able to prop them up. That is, if I hadn't been squandering my income chasing those elusive winners.

Much as I used to convince myself that I would hit a winning streak with gambling, I was certain myself that the housing market would pick up and my racehorses might one day come good. I was at Derby County at the time, my fifth club, and I was one of the highest paid players in the game at the time. But it wasn't enough to bail me out. I raised money from loans from the bank by using the three signing-on payments of my new contract. When the payments were due, the club would pay them to the bank instead of to me. In order to facilitate this, the club had to be notified, and that alerted them to my financial worries. It was all getting very messy.

I left Derby County in 1992 and became player-manager and eventually manager of Plymouth Argyle. After a successful season in my second year, I ended up leaving due to circumstances which were a result of my gambling and my messy financial situation. This was a massive disappointment to me as I always felt I had what it took to be a great manager. As it was, I never got back into management and I think this was due to my gambling. When my businesses started suffering at the end of my football career, I eventually had to have an IVA, an Individual Voluntary Arrangement to deal with my debts.

I had one last challenge – I wanted to get 1,000 league appearances. And I did, after playing two games for Bolton at the age of 46. One was 80 minutes at Stoke when I came on after our goalkeeper Aidan Davison got sent off. I had a very good game and, because of that, Bruce Rioch played me against Wolves in the first leg of the play-off semi-final to a capacity crowd at Molineux. We lost 2–1 but, to this day, I get people saying how well I played that day. Bolton won the second leg 2–0 and went on to gain promotion to what is now the Premier League. West Ham and their manager, Harry Redknapp, wanted me as a goalkeeping cover, but I never played in the first team and eventually joined Leyton Orient to play seven games and reaching a record 1,005 league appearances. My football career was all but over.

I spoke with ex-Chelsea and Manchester United manager, Tommy Docherty, and he recommended that I got onto the after-dinner speaking circuit. He told me how much I would enjoy it and that he thought I would be good at it – especially as a motivational speaker. He told me that I should seriously consider it, rather than hanging around in the forlorn hope of another role in management. He told me he was doing three or four speaking events a week and it was proving lucrative but also very satisfying work without any of the pressures of being in football. I decided to give it a go. It was, at first, harder than I thought and I didn't have such good nights to begin with. But I grew quickly into the role and became more assured and confident. I also managed to develop other contracts mostly in the football world. After a while I started to build a terrific reputation as an entertaining speaker, and that was when I decided that this was the best future for me.

Of course, it was at one of these engagements that I met Steph for the first time. It was the start of a new chapter in my life but one that came with clouds. I had, by then, been gambling for years and it had filled the space left in my life by football. It continued to have a devastating effect on my life. When I met Steph, this was still my dark little secret. Something had to change.

STEPH'S STORY

In early 2013 we moved from my little two-bedroomed house in Colchester to Mersea Island. It's a place I used to visit with my parents as a child, so I had a great affinity with the island and some lovely memories. It is also the place I took Pete on our first date. It's a tiny island in Essex tucked away in the Blackwater and Colne Estuaries. Mersea Island is renowned for its oysters. They have been harvested off the island since Roman times and are now shipped across the world. It has quaint beaches, fresh fish and seafood and, most importantly, it gave Pete and I the ability to lead a private life. The locals seemed friendly and respectful about Pete's need for privacy. It was the perfect choice for us. We both relished a healthy lifestyle so fresh local produce, long beach walks for exercise and the rustic, coastal lifestyle was everything we were looking for.

I hoped this would be a fresh start but gambling still had a grip on Pete. At this point, I guess my life had also become a double life too. I was now working 50–70 hours a week, knowing Pete would be at home gambling. It started to become the norm.

In 2014, Pete was working in India for three weeks as a pundit for the World Cup. During this time his bank statement arrived in the post. Normally this is something he would have scooped up and squirreled away as he was very seasoned in keeping his finances well hidden. This time, I was the first one to see it land on the doormat.

There I sat holding the envelope. I felt excited that, finally, my investigation could be concluded with the knowledge of what was inside the envelope. I finally had the chance to see Pete's true financial position. But for three days I held off opening it, leaving it on the mantle above the fireplace, wrestling with my conscience. I was riddled with guilt, knowing that opening it was a terrible thing for me to do. A betrayal of trust. At the same time, I knew that I needed to know the extent of his illness.

Eventually, with trembling hands, I opened it to find pages and pages of transactions. It was the previous month's statement from his main bank account. And the records clearly showed large sums of money being paid to a betting company. I used a calculator to add up how much he had lost to them. In that month alone it was just over £18,000. I asked myself, if he was able to lose that amount in just *one* month, how much had he lost in total over the years? Physically I felt faint and, honestly, I thought I might be sick. The shock and reality hit me like a bolt of lightning.

I rang Missy and she visited me straight away. I asked her to check if my calculations were correct as I was in disbelief. She told me that I was right. It was heartbreaking seeing the anguish on her face. The last thing I wanted to do was alarm Missy and burden her with this problem, but at that moment there was full exposure of the challenge I was facing. She advised me that I should keep my financial affairs and accounts separate from Pete's. It must have been a very concerning time for Missy, huge alarm bells must have gone off for her. I was in such shock that I started to have a panic attack. I just didn't know what to do. How was I going to handle this? What should I tell Pete? And how would I explain opening his confidential post?

I still had time before Pete was due to return and those weeks gave me the time to get my head around things. Reality had hit me, and I understood that he seriously needed help and that his addiction was severe. I knew Pete's username – I'd seen it one day when Pete's laptop screen was open whilst he popped to the toilet – and I emailed the betting company. I begged the gambling company for help. I made them aware of Pete's serious addiction. I even gave them his user ID so that they would know exactly who I was talking about. They emailed me back to tell me that, due to data protection, they couldn't discuss the problem with me and suggested that I contact Gamblers Anonymous. I've since learned that they did nothing to action my email. I knew Pete would never sit with a stranger and talk about addiction, especially as he couldn't even admit it to himself at that time – as he was still in complete denial. I knew I couldn't speak to his GP for help or his bank. There was literally no one who would help.

Pete returned from India. I wasn't intending on confronting him, but I really couldn't hold it in, so I calmly told him what I'd found. He was, quite rightly, cross – furious with me for opening his mail. I think it was because I had finally cracked into his secret world and there was no way of wriggling out. He refused to talk about it and turned it round to me being in the wrong for interfering in his business. He was still very much in denial, but I had opened the fortress door, now I needed to crack through the wall and get Pete to realise he needed help.

Life was becoming ever more difficult for me. I was living with a chronic gambler, I had a very demanding job and I was having to put on a front for my dear friends and family. I felt such guilt hiding it from them as I'd always had such close, loving relationships with them all. I had always been able to be completely open and honest with them so having to keep something secret was such an enormous burden on me.

Around a month after this revelation, we had an horrendous experience. I was in my early forties and thought I was starting to go through the menopause. But Pete was convinced I was showing signs of pregnancy. One evening I woke up in the middle of the night in absolute agony with terrible lower abdomen pain. Pete helped me to the bathroom where I suffered a horrendous complete miscarriage. Whilst waiting for the paramedics, Pete was amazing, keeping me calm, kissing and holding me. The paramedics arrived but we felt that we couldn't go to hospital for fear of Pete being recognised and the press finding out. For us, this was a deeply private and personal situation. So, the paramedics gave me pain relief and kindly stayed with us until the pain and bleeding started to subside.

For the next three to four days Pete nursed me day and night. He was amazing and attentive which, for a man his age, I felt was wonderful and this helped me to emotionally and physically recover. Pete didn't leave me alone and, strangely enough, I noticed he didn't gamble once. I knew then that he could quit for me. From our sad loss I gained hope for the first time. The gambling wasn't Pete. The real Pete was the one with me now.

From then on, I found a different mindset. I decided to separate the addiction from the man. You must remember addicts suppress their conscience. In fact, I think they lose their conscience. Pete would always find ways of getting money. He could lie and be devious, but I never took it personally. It's part of the horrible, nasty disease.

The twelve months leading up to Pete finally quitting in 2015, did become intolerable. It was all coming to a head. I felt I had nowhere to turn but I knew that, if I left him, not only would I have failed in my promise to his dad, but that Pete would literally have nothing and nobody. The fear of him committing suicide kept creeping in. I would have loved to have been able to talk to people in a similar situation and unload my feelings but, living with the addict, you become the forgotten and silent victim. I distanced myself from family and friends which obviously made me feel more isolated. Knowing what I do now, I should never have felt shame and embarrassment in telling my friends and family. Without a doubt, they would have been there for me but, at the time, I was locked into the world of gambling addiction.

I guess I started to see if I could change Pete's mindset too. At times when he looked strained I would tell him he could talk to me about anything and there was nothing we couldn't sort out together. I tried to give him the trust and confidence to open up to me. I tried to get him engaged in our dreams of the future and reminded him that, whilst he was still gambling, they could never be fulfilled. I also made an effort to use the word "lose" daily in conversation.

By Christmas 2014, Pete's gambling problem was really taking a hold. He was starting to look gaunt and quite ill. The house we were living in at the time had a large main lounge and a smaller adjoining sitting room and it was there that Pete was now spending almost all his time – watching the racing. iPhones were now all the rage, so he no longer needed the laptop, everything he needed to gamble was on his phone. So, we were back where we started. Mobile phone in one hand, TV remote control in the other.

I wanted to come up with a special Christmas present for Pete – something romantic. I felt we both needed a break away as he had become more and more withdrawn by now and I was increasingly worried about his health. I thought it would be lovely after all our hard work for us to get away and have some quality time alone. I planned it all – booking top restaurants and beautiful hotels that I thought we would both really like. I organised two nights in the heart of Cambridge and a third night in the centre of Newmarket just a few miles away. I had planned on us spending time having leisurely lunches, sightseeing and generally having a wonderful time together. It may sound strange that I decided to take him to Newmarket, but I had checked that there was no race meeting that day and, deep down, I also hoped the home of horse racing would spur him into opening up about his addiction. I honestly thought this would be the perfect start to the new year and that Pete would love it as we had always loved travelling together.

On Christmas morning, I handed him an envelope and he opened it to find all the exciting details about what I had planned for the break. To my dismay his face didn't light up as I had expected. In fact, I could see he was disappointed. My heart sank. He wasn't impressed. I put it down to the fact that he was feeling low, and that this reaction just reflected his recent depressed state. I truly thought that the break away would help him.

New Year's Day arrived, and Pete grudgingly loaded the car with our cases. I kept being upbeat to keep the mood positive. I was certain he would enjoy it once we got there. Arriving in Cambridge was lovely. It was so pretty with Christmas decorations and twinkling trees. What a beautiful city. The university colleges, churches and stunning architecture are steeped in history. Everything was idyllic. I thought it was stunning and the stay would be a special way for us to start the new year. But, after two days in Cambridge, Pete was becoming more and more agitated by the minute. It was clear to me that he definitely wasn't happy. I couldn't seem to get him engaged in anything. I was now starting to feel really concerned as Pete was showing signs of real mental health illness.

When we arrived at our next destination, Newmarket, Pete's behaviour was even worse. I couldn't understand it. I knew he was betting on his iPhone via his account so what was the problem? I finally broke and said, "Shall we just go home, it's obvious you don't want to be here." I was shattered. I'd had good intentions of giving Pete a lovely treat, but it had all become so miserable. His response was, "Yes, I want to go home. Going away for New Year is not what I ever would want to do." We began packing to go home. I demanded to know what was so wrong with having a New Year's break. He dropped his head and told me that New Year's Day is one of the biggest days of the year for horse racing. I then realised that, for him, I had totally messed up. I had interrupted his pattern of betting. Now I could see that, deep down, he was furious with me. We left in silence. I cried some of the way home. It was the first time I had cried over his gambling in front of him. The silence remained in the car all the way back to Mersea Island. I was so terribly hurt.

I now had proof that the addict has no conscience at all. The only thing that drives them is the drug — in Pete's case, gambling — and they concentrate on getting rid of anything that gets in the way of that. It didn't cross Pete's mind that he had hurt me and that was heartbreaking. As difficult as it was, on that occasion, I had to keep reminding myself that it was the illness and not the man causing me pain. I doubled my efforts to get Pete back. That incident gave me the confidence to start using the word "lose" even more. I was now at war with that blasted betting company. Every time they whispered "win" in Pete's ear, I'd be there to say "lose". They were never going to beat me.

CHAPTER 8

THE GRAND FINAL

STEPH'S STORY

I knew Pete was capable of turning his back on gambling as he had shown that resolve after my miscarriage. I knew I had to be patient and stay calm, but the situation was becoming intolerable. Everything we talked about, our future and our dreams, was at stake. I kept pushing the positives and hoped that he was getting a mental picture of how happily we could live without gambling. I really think he began to listen and understand this, but the gambling had such a tight hold on him. I didn't want to put extra pressure on him. I knew applying pressure, laying blame and making ultimatums were the worst things I could do. It would make the illness worse.

I could see that Pete's health was now becoming affected. Eight weeks into the new year he had obviously had a very heavy loss and his mood was still extremely low. He had not been engaging in normal family life since the New Year and now he seemed completely obsessed with the horse racing. It was now starting to affect my own well-being and I was beginning to emotionally detach myself from Pete. I knew he had noticed my mood change. I started to look up smaller houses for sale, leaving the web pages open on the laptop in the hope he would see it and worry that I was preparing to move out and buy somewhere else. I felt I had nothing left in my resource toolbox to pull out in a bid to get him out of this hole. In my desperation I thought that maybe, if he thought he was losing me, he might just see sense. Eventually, I very calmly told him I wanted to spend a few nights in the spare room, something I had never done before. He looked at me sadly and said, "OK." Deep down it broke my heart to hurt him, but I could see the addiction had brought him to his lowest point. The next morning, I went downstairs. Pete was in the lounge and he looked ghastly, absolutely horrendous. I could see he hadn't slept a wink all night. He said: "I need to talk to you. I have something to say." I stood frozen in the middle of the lounge. He said, "If I don't quit gambling, your next move will be out the front door. I'm going to lose you and I can't let that happen. I'm going to quit but I know I'm going to need your help." I burst into tears and said, "You're never going to lose me and of course I'll help you because we're going to get through this together."

We stood there holding each other so tightly, crying. Pete's nickname for me is "Titch" as I'm so much smaller than him. He towered above me and I felt his sheer weight fall into me. Pete's physique is amazing for his age, so it felt like a ton of weight was falling from his body. It was as though 45 years of strain left his body – it was quite a remarkable feeling. We were both forced down on the sofa by the weight of his relief – both in floods of tears. It was one of the greatest moments of my life. I knew, at that moment, he was going to stop and that was the biggest win of his life. And I knew that I had won. That vile betting company had lost.

Pete asked me to give up work to help him through the ordeal and I knew that it was the only way it would work. I had to be there for him 100 per cent of the time or the temptation for him to gamble would be too much. We needed to work on this 24/7. I knew the sacrifice I was making would be very difficult for me. I was walking away from a much-loved career, but I was more than willing to make that sacrifice for the man I loved. I was the only one who could help him recover and we would do it together. I also knew that, even though it would be tight financially, we would find a way. We had to take one day at a time. We had to build a whole new life for Pete as his routine had been thrown upside down.

In the first week I was really shocked to see Pete suffering with full blown physical withdrawal symptoms – no different to that of an alcoholic or drug addict. Without his usual day-to-day structure, he was at a complete loss. He couldn't concentrate and he was extremely irritable and very jittery. On the third night he suffered night sweats and horrendous insomnia. I suggested he took a diazepam tablet which he had previously been prescribed for a muscle injury. In that first week he had no appetite and he lost weight.

I planned nice things to do to keep his mind occupied. I suggested each morning that we take our poodle, Charlie Buttons, for a long walk along the beach near our home to set the tone for the day. We tried to go out for lunch that week but halfway through the meal Pete got irritable and wanted to go home. I ensured that I remained calm and understanding as I could see he had bad withdrawal symptoms. I would comfort him and tell him he was strong enough to get through this. I knew I was his backbone and I realised I had to be the strongest out of the two of us. I remained patient and positive with him and even when he became irritated. At times he would try to pick arguments with me, but I didn't take it personally or rise to it. I understood why he was doing it and I ignored it. I knew it was just a symptom of his withdrawal. After about three months Pete's extreme withdrawal behaviour started to gradually settle down. Pete was able to stay out longer and he became less distracted. I could sense he was beginning to come through. He really was far more relaxed both physically and mentally.

Only a few months after Pete quit we received a phone call from Leicester Infirmary Hospital telling us that Pete's dad had suffered a major stroke and he was at the end of his life. I knew this would devastate Pete as he adored his father. We drove straight to the hospital and Pete asked me if I would go in with him to see his dad for the last time. I don't think he felt he could cope on his own, which is totally understandable. We stood either side of the bed, each holding one of Les's hands. The stroke had been severe, but he was able to communicate with us. With tears running from my eyes, I said to Les, "He's done it. He's really done it, he's quit." I could see that Les understood and I could see his relief. I had fulfilled my promise. Les sadly died a few hours later but passed away knowing Pete was no longer a gambling addict. I was worried Pete might relapse at that time but fortunately he didn't. I think he also wanted to stay free of gambling to honour his dad's memory. He found the inner strength to stay on the right path.

Six months into Pete's recovery we set the date for our wedding. The dream was starting to come true. Pete's subscription to the *Racing Post* had been cancelled but we still got other newspapers which at times had horse racing coverage in the middle section. I would always remove these pages. One morning Pete watched me as I took out the racing section from the day's paper and said: "Steph, you really don't need to do that anymore." It was so lovely, but I still had a little nagging worry that somehow the urge to bet would overpower him. If I walked into the room and he innocently switched the TV channel over my stomach lurched in fear that he had been watching horse racing. I had to learn to trust him. I realised that I had also been affected by the gambling experience and had my own recovery to make. I had to remain psychologically tough.

During that first year, I encouraged him to do as many things as possible to keep himself busy and his mind occupied. We would play golf together and this would become a wonderful release for him. It helped immensely and he got more and more into it. After that year, Pete's irritability ebbed away and his mood swings were less and less frequent. It was wonderful to see that his love of football was returning. He used to watch football on TV and kept spotting problems with the current goalkeepers. He would point out that certain effective techniques weren't being used. I suggested that he write them down and that's when the *Shilton's Secrets* videos were produced to explore Pete's fourteen basic techniques that modern day goalkeepers were missing. Pete loved working on this project and felt it was truly part of his legacy. I contacted St George's Park, the FA's national football centre and left a message for the England goalkeeping trainer to ask if he would like to meet Pete to discuss the project and Pete's interest in supporting him with his wealth of goalkeeping experience. I honestly thought the trainer would be ecstatic at the suggestion but, to my surprise, I received a message back saying that he didn't want to meet Pete. Basically, it was "Thanks, but no thanks." If there was ever a time when Pete may have fallen off the wagon it was then. It was such an insult and a huge knock-back. At the time, I was so worried about how the rejection would affect him. But Pete was now the new Pete, and he just shrugged his shoulders and moved on. I'm still aghast as to why you would turn down the opportunity to get guidance from one of the greatest goalkeepers in the world. Surely they should welcome and want his amazing expertise. I think the issue is that many coaches feel threatened by Pete's history and experience in the game.

I'd given up my job, but I told Pete I didn't want to ever be a kept woman – I was far too independent. So, between us, we came up with the idea of setting up our own company, Peter & Steffi Shilton Consultancy

Ltd. I didn't want to waste my health care and management expertise and found I was able to transfer those skills to our business. Before long, I was looking after Pete's diary and working on events for him. I basically ran his career. It was important that we had a joint project, and we took it very seriously, getting expert advice and drawing up extensive business plans. I felt this was also vital for Pete's recovery and it was important also that he was involved in the finances so we could begin to build trust. It became a great success and something we both really enjoyed setting up and working on. Pete is still in demand globally. It's quite astonishing that after 50 plus years he is still involved in football. After a while, I also returned to do some freelance NHS work, but I had to tread carefully as I was worried Pete might lapse if I wasn't around. But, ultimately, Pete never let me down and I built my trust in him. We both had to work hard but we were now looking forward to a new future together – finally coming out of the darkness into the dawn.

PETE'S STORY

Just before I met Steph, I had been single for a while and was set in my gambling routine. I honestly could not see a life without gambling. I was forever chasing big wins. Just before we met I had a brilliant run and was up £20,000 on my betting account. I was on such a high. Now, most people would say, "Time to withdraw the money from the account and bank it, Shilts" but – oh no – not me. I wanted another win – a bigger win. I was on a roll. But you know what I'm going to say, don't you? Yes, the money disappeared into losses within days. By trying to win more, I lost it all. I was really depressed as I knew I'd blown a huge chance to bank a really large sum of money. At that time gambling had become the main preoccupation of my life. Only when I worked did I get any distraction from it. I was living on my own, so I had the freedom to stay up most of the night betting after an afternoon online.

One of the best evening's work I have ever done is when I spoke at the Rotary Club dinner and met Steph. From the moment Steph entered my life, I felt better about myself and about life in general. It was like I had this little ray of warm light enter into my dark world. Falling in love with Steph was so easy but hiding my secret world of gambling was so difficult. I knew I could experience great highs in our relationship, and

I knew we had a chance of a brilliant future together, but I also knew, as loving as Steph is, that financial security is highly important to her. Commitment and financial stability, for her, went hand in hand. This all made me start to feel very uncomfortable.

I tried to be secretive about my addiction and finances and the longer the relationship went on, the more I knew my insecurity would grow. I needed time to work things out so as not to lose Steph. How on earth could I tell her the truth about it all? Surely, the truth would mean she would leave me. Deep down, I was slowly feeling more and more embarrassed, but I was still gambling. Towards the end I knew I just couldn't go on living that way. But, after a lifetime of gambling, how could I ever be free from it? I was completely in pieces.

As Steph explained, things started to come to a head when she opened the bank statement. She probably didn't realise at the time, but I wasn't really angry at *her* but at myself because my secret had been exposed. It was a reality check, and it wasn't appreciated. Around six months before I quit, that uncomfortable, insecure feeling was becoming more and more intense. The gambling had complete control over me. I was trapped in a vicious cycle of constantly chasing a win and losing. I felt that I really needed the big win so Steph and I could have everything we dreamed of. I really longed for Steph to be my wife and I loved the thought of it, but I just knew that while I couldn't be financially stable she would never enter into a marriage with me. The word "lose" kept popping into my head – *lose, lose, lose*. I think this was Steph's tactics working on my mindset.

The possibility of losing Steph was becoming very real. In fact, it was becoming a genuine fear. I was turning more and more into myself, feeling like I was slowly sinking into quicksand. It was mid-February, and I was still desperately chasing wins. I felt stuck, like I was wading waist high in mud. I was seriously struggling. It felt like I was living in a bad dream and Steph was drifting further away from me. The loneliness and isolation were truly setting in and I couldn't see a way out.

I found myself, one Friday night in a godforsaken nightmare of a routine, sitting in my small TV room, mobile phone on one side of me, remote control on the other. But something in me was changing. This routine was no longer making me happy. In fact, it now had me in a state of pure misery. What the hell was I chasing? Why was I living like this?

Friday and Saturday came and went and, before I knew it, I had wasted yet another weekend on nothing but losses. Steph was ever more distant, it was now really starting to hit me, I was facing nothing but losses. Despite this, I did the only thing I knew how to do: try and win back all that I had lost over the weekend. But I had lost literally all my disposable funds before Sunday even came around.

In pure desperation, while Steph was in the kitchen cooking Sunday lunch, I sneaked upstairs, through our bedroom and into the en suite with my mobile phone where I thought I couldn't be heard. I telephoned an agent who I was also friends with and asked him to fast track payment for a job I had done the previous week. In my industry, you tend to get paid a week or two after an event, but I asked if he could pay me immediately. He agreed. I can't explain the anxiety you feel, as an addict, when you hit a bad run of losses. The desperation for money is a terrible feeling. When the agent didn't bat an eyelid and agreed to transfer the payment, my entire body went from being rigid with tensity to filled with sheer physical relief. I took a deep breath to relax and looked into the wall mirror in front of me to see Steph's reflection. She'd been standing behind me, in the doorway of the bedroom. Her eyes were filled with tears and she was ashen-faced. I could tell she had heard the entire conversation and was clearly horrified at my desperation. I dropped my head in shame as she silently walked out and back downstairs. My heart just sank, and fear ran through me. My life was in tatters. Somewhere deep down, I realised that I was losing everything, including the most important thing in my life – my Steph.

We ate dinner in complete silence. I just didn't know what to say to Steph and denial was no longer an option, we were beyond that. Later that day, Steph came into my TV room and told me she had decided to move into the spare room for a few nights. My heart sank as I looked into those African almond eyes of hers that I had fallen in love with a few years before. I could see her pain and her hurt. Finally, I saw what this wretched gambling life was doing and destroying. I knew then, without a doubt, that I was breaking her heart. Why had I not seen what I was doing to her before? I was so tangled up in this blasted world of gambling that I had been blind to what I was destroying. How could I have not seen this?

Steph not wanting to share the bedroom with me was a signal that something was drastically wrong. the only time we weren't together was when I was working abroad and, even then, we hated not sleeping together – we literally hated every minute of it. We'd count the hours down until I would be back home. We always agreed that couples that sleep apart always end up living apart. At that moment, I really believed that this was the start of her leaving me. I could clearly see that she was reaching the end. My little ray of sunshine had started to disappear.

I left Steph alone that night. I didn't want to rock the boat any more than I had done. I tossed and turned all night. I knew how much she loved me. There and then, I knew I couldn't lose her, so the gambling had to go. It was as though a light bulb just turned on in my head. For several months, thoughts had been whirling around in my head. I was beginning to realise I was gaining nothing but misery with the gambling. And at that moment it had come to a head. Then and there, I could clearly see it for what it was, and the word "lose" was now spinning in my head. The only way out of all this was to walk away from the gambling. I made the decision, but little did I know that the battle had only just started. My entire life would have to change to be free from gambling…

THE SECOND HALF

CHAPTER 9

DREAMS COME TRUE

PETE'S STORY

I never thought of myself as a romantic. I'm not much of an emotional type – more like the strong, silent type. I like going out for meals with Steph and have been known to buy her roses on occasions. But I wasn't like that until I met Steph so maybe she brought it out in me. I knew I wanted to marry Steph, so it wasn't too long before I popped the question. But I didn't plan the proposal, it was an impromptu spur of the moment act. I must admit I felt a touch of fear, a few seconds of apprehension. What if she said no? I had been pretty sure she wanted to marry me, but you never know until you ask. It would have been pretty demoralising if she had turned me down. I wanted to make our wedding day something special so, when we got engaged, I told Steph, "I want you to have a white wedding in a church, it's what you've always wanted, so you will have it."

And it was a beautiful wedding. It took place in a lovely spot on Mersea Island, where Steph had grown up. On the 10th of December 2016 about 150 guests attended the church service, at St Paul's Church in West Mersea. Our guests included *Coronation Street* veteran Bill Roache, who plays Ken Barlow. We had met Bill at a charity event and had become friends – he's such a nice fellow. Despite his busy workload he said he would be delighted to come, and he made it down from Manchester. That's the sort of guy he is. Another guest was *MasterChef* presenter, Greg Wallace. Again, Greg is someone I met through charity work and became friends with. Greg was filming *MasterChef* abroad at the time so there was no knowing if he would make it. But, like Bill, he took the trouble to find a way. He couldn't stay long as he had to fly off the next morning to film the final of the cooking show, but it was lovely of him to have got there at all. Greg loves his football, he's a big supporter of Millwall and also follows Spurs. Also in attendance was former professional boxer, John H. Stracey. I'd always been a big admirer of John as a world champion boxer.

Retired sprint athlete, Derek Redmond, who took part in *Total Wipe Out* with me was there. No one will ever forget what he achieved 25 years ago when he fell to his knees during the 400m after tearing his hamstring. Applauded and encouraged by the 65,000 people in the stadium, Derek hobbled to the finish line with the help of his father, Jim, who defied security and bolted onto the track to aid his son across the line. Jockey, Bob Champion OBE whom I met at a local charity event was there and, again, he is such a nice man. He had a great time at the wedding. Steph's uncle and aunt, funnily enough, are members at Newmarket and they enjoy a day out at the races. So it was apt for them to be seated next to Bob and his wife at our wedding reception.

Actor, Jess Conrad MBE also attended along with his wife. I'd known Jess for a few years after we met up at a golf day, and he has become a dear friend of ours. You just wouldn't think he is in his 80s when he looks no more than 60. He's such a laugh, and he seems to have done it all in his career – both music and films. Who he doesn't know isn't worth knowing! It was a pity Ray Clemence and Gary Lineker were unable to attend, but they were both invited.

Because of my footballing history and our guest list, some of the celebrity magazines wanted to be involved. While they do pay very well, we didn't want them taking over the wedding with their own photographers. We just wanted it to be quiet and intimate. With this in mind, we asked our guests not to take pictures on the day as we had arranged professional photographers to be around for the whole day and the evening to take pictures. We intended to make the photographs available as a gift to our guests. They had free access to all of these so they could select those they wanted to keep to remember the day. We got permission from Reverend Sam, who married us, for our photographer to position himself right in the corner, at the front and near the altar. I wanted a picture of Steph walking up the aisle in her white dress.

Steph organised both the service and the reception and she loved doing it. Around 70 guests were invited to the ceremony with an extra

70 guests expected at the evening reception at Hintlesham Hall, an estate in Suffolk. Guests were invited to stay there for two nights, the night before the reception and one after courtesy of myself and Steph. The evening before the wedding I stayed at home only five minutes from the church. Steph stayed with her bridesmaids at the venue which had been the location of our first date. That must have been special for her. I hired a vintage Bentley to take me to the church, and it took about two minutes to drive me up the road.

Being a singer, Steph arranged all the music for our church service. She didn't want me to know any of the songs she had chosen. My only input was choosing the hymns to be sung by the choir. The service was filled with beautiful songs, but my biggest surprise came just before the reading. Steph had arranged for a Welsh tenor to be hidden in the choir. Suddenly he walked out to the altar, looked straight at me and sang Luciano Pavarotti's greatest hit and the theme tune to Italia '90, "Nessun Dorma". I don't think there was a dry eye in the church, including mine. It was moment that gave me goosebumps. A great surprise.

Another highlight of the service was a reading by Bill Roache of a poem that Steph had written. Even Bill choked up a bit as he read it – it was so emotional. I found out later that when Steph sent her poem to Bill he told her he had a tear in his eye as he first read it. That is typical of Steph, though. When she sits down to do something, when she makes up her mind, she makes sure she does it properly. There were some that told us afterwards that they couldn't believe Steph had actually written the poem. It was so beautiful and summed up our journey together. So many people in the congregation told us how moving the whole ceremony had been for them.

The evening buffet was laid out on a giant table designed to look like a football pitch with a goal at either end. The chef based the buffet menu on football stadium food – hot pies, burgers and chips – all delicious treats you would get at Wembley on a match day. We had a big brass band, all dressed in war uniforms. We had organised a singer for the evening who, unfortunately, was taken ill shortly before the wedding. We were thrilled that Steve Collazo, the former lead singer from Odyssey, took his place and he was excellent. He certainly got the dancing going and brought the party to life. Graham Jolly, the famous mind reader and magician performed at our reception dinner. His performance was mind blowing and fabulous. He did a great trick with a wonderful friend of mine, Andrew Breakwell, one of the finest divorce solicitors in the country. Graham made Andrew's watch disappear from around his very wrist and even though Andrew has an excellent legal brain I doubt if he could work out how he managed that.

My best man was my dear friend, Lloyd Scott. Lloyd was once a goalkeeper but is now a charity fundraiser, best known for his charity marathons. He competed in the 2002 London Marathon in a deep-sea diving costume. Lloyd introduced himself to me when I was playing in a game for Nottingham Forest against Chelsea. He played for Orient and got into the England youth squad, before joining Watford briefly before moving on to Blackpool and making his league debut. After a short spell at Blackpool, he returned to Essex to play for Dagenham in the GM Vauxhall Conference. Lloyd is quite a unique man. In 1987 he was working in the fire service and rescued two children from a blaze. He was admitted to hospital for smoke inhalation. During some routine tests they found he had leukaemia. Lloyd was in Hammersmith Hospital whilst I was visiting with the England squad including Gary Lineker, Bryan Robson and Peter Beardsley. We were preparing for a World Cup qualifying match against Poland at that time.

Lloyd was the subject of an episode of the biographical show *This Is Your Life* and a recipient of the big red book. I was on holiday in Portugal when it was being screened, but I flew back on my own just to appear on the programme to honour him. The show makers surprised him by initially played a video of me wishing him well and saying I couldn't make it because I was on holiday. I then appeared from backstage to surprise him. He couldn't believe I had cut short my holiday. It was the least I could do for such a good friend.

Lloyd was a great best man for me, but he did give me a scare on the morning of the wedding. When I woke up and I went downstairs and couldn't find him. I shouted out for him but there was no reply. I couldn't find him anywhere in the house. I thought that the pressure had got to him and that he had done a runner. I needn't have worried as he then walked through the front door having just popped out to the local shop to pick up smoked salmon, orange juice and a newspaper for me.

I later discovered that Steph and Lloyd had been plotting behind my back to find some stories to tell about me in his Best Man's speech. Steph contacted my old teammate, Tony Woodcock in search of some "locker room funnies" as she calls them. Lloyd told a story during his speech about my time at Nottingham Forest that Steph thinks is hilarious. When I first signed for Forest I would always turn up clean and smart, even for training, as I had always taken great pride in myself. Unbeknown to me, the lads would start bantering about this behind my back. I always felt I should be immaculate to set standards but obviously it was providing the lads with a giggle and fed into their usual mickey-taking. They had noticed that I always turned up with a big sports bag and I would neatly fold all my gear into it even after the end of a game or training session. Once, while I was having a debriefing with Cloughie, they decided to have a laugh. Whilst I was out of the room, they hid two extremely heavy dumb-bells that they had taken from the gym and planted them under my neatly folded gear in my bag, then they waited for me to come back into the changing room. I picked up the bag, threw it over one of my shoulders and casually walked out saying, "See you all tomorrow, lads." According to Tony, you could have heard a pin drop in that changing room. They vowed never to take the mickey out of me again and realised they had a man of steel between the posts. I've never admitted it until now, but the bag *did* seem a tad heavier than usual.

The whole wedding day was wonderful – it really was perfect. It was one of the most beautiful days of my life and I was determined to make the honeymoon something really special too, something that we would remember for the rest of our lives. And it was. To this very day, we never tire of recalling our honeymoon moments.

At the time, I was worried that Steph's fear of flying and the fact that she had never flown long haul before, only short flights. Barbados was, of course, a long-haul flight. But in anticipation of this, Steph took a Fear of Flying course which completely cured all her anxieties. The course began with mock flight to start with, followed a short, real flight where they would fake turbulence and make a few unusual movements. The course helped assure those fearful of flying how sophisticated and adaptable modern planes are. We also took a short flight to Newquay where the pilot took her into the cockpit and showed her the auto-pilot button that, when pressed, would safely land the small plane back at the airport. Steph gained her certificate by taking that course and now receives loads of support whenever she flies. And I needn't have worried because Steph thoroughly enjoyed every minute of the flight to Barbados.

We stayed at The Colony Club, a lovely five-star resort. One night we were enjoying a nightcap in the bar. Steph had her usual cocktail and I had a brandy. There was a two-piece band including a girl singer. They struck up a Caribbean song "Kingston Town" by UB40 and we started to dance. Yes, I was in the mood for dancing, and we danced for three or four songs before we sat down back at the bar. Suddenly we became aware that people were clapping. I had been a contestant on *Strictly Come Dancing* in 2010, before I met Steph. I've said on numerous occasions that I would definitely have done better if Steph had been in my life then. She loves to dance and is a great mover. We enjoy dancing together, it's a great love of ours. That was one of the most romantic moments imaginable. It was certainly the most romantic moment of my life, a moment of magic I have never tired of recounting. I'll never forget the lyrics to "Kingston Town", whenever I hear those words, it reminds me of Barbados and being lost in the dance with my bride.

STEPH'S STORY

Pete had been free of his gambling addiction for a year by the Christmas of 2015, so the new year seemed the perfect time to start planning our future together and to make commitments. He had turned a corner with his withdrawal symptoms and our wedding was one of the dreams that we could now make come true. We had something special to look forward to.

We did much of the planning together which, after everything we had been through together, seemed the right thing to do. I'm a devout Christian so I wanted not just a glamorous wedding but one with true depth and meaning. We attended couple's classes at the church and heard our bans being read at every service. I was so serious about saying my vows in front God – it meant so much to me as it would mean that our marriage would be blessed.

One thing we didn't do together was choose my wedding dress. Obviously, I wanted this to be a secret and Pete knew nothing about it.

I chose a beautiful dress from Italy — full length and slinky, with crystal buttons down the back. Apparently, the number of buttons on the dress represents the number of years your marriage will last. There were 27 on mine!

With my musical background I wanted the ceremony to feature striking music. Pete left that side of things to me and he focused on organising the cars and the logistics of the day. I wanted to give Pete a special wedding gift so, secretly, I contacted a Welsh tenor, John Pierce. I arranged prior to the wedding to meet John at the church where I told him I wanted him to sing "Nessun Dorma" especially for Pete. He sang it for me that day at the church — his amazing vocals bouncing off the walls and ceiling. It was so magical that it made me cry. I knew how special it would be on the day. Just before we took our vows, John, who had been wearing a robe so he looked like he was just a member of the choir, took off the robe to reveal a tux. He walked out to the front of the congregation and sang. Many men in the church were reduced to tears and Peter was utterly amazed. He just looked at me and said, "Thank you."

Typical of me, I was so nervous on the day of the wedding. I was used to performing in front of people, but this was something so emotional and special to me that it got my stomach turning. We knelt at the high altar and received our blessing. I remember thinking that everything in our life was going to start from here. Everything else was in the past. Addicted gamblers have only one dream and that is the big win, nothing else excites them. But I knew that this was *our* big win. Our ultimate dream was getting married and so our first dream had come true. We had worked so hard in getting to this point that I wanted it to be perfect.

Beforehand, we had an awful lot of interest from newspapers and magazines in covering the wedding but we both agreed that our special day was off limits to the media. We wanted it to be a personal and private day and so we turned down all the offers. We were happy to give the press a photo that was released on the day. Some press had turned up outside the church but there were also many locals who had gathered to wish us well, which was lovely. They were all so amazing and kind to us on the day. There's a lovely cafe opposite the church and they offered a special wedding breakfast for their customers. I really wanted to involve everyone on the island, and I was happy that our local businesses benefitted.

Pete looked so handsome dressed in his morning suit. He had been awarded an OBE, but he is so modest and unassuming that he never wears the medal. He would be too worried that people would think he was showing off. But I knew how proud he was of it, so I really wanted him to wear it at the wedding. I told him: "You must wear it in the church, Pete. It's an honour you've been given." And that was the only time he has ever worn it and is ever likely to.

The vicar had told Pete that he mustn't look round when I walked down the aisle, but he couldn't help himself. He watched me from the moment I walked into the church until I reached his side. I'm so pleased he did. I felt so special when he whispered, "You look so beautiful."

Pete gave a speech at the wedding reception at Hintlesham Hall. He said that I had turned his life around. He started to become emotional, and I started cuddling him as I knew that paying tribute to me was his way of saying thank you. Our guests obviously had no idea the extent of the journey we had come on. Our wedding day meant so much more than becoming Mr & Mrs – for us it was also a celebration of our union, what we'd achieved together. We knew that, by standing together, there was nothing we couldn't achieve.

Our honeymoon was one of the dreams that we had had to put on hold until Pete's financial situation had improved. I didn't want to get into debt over it. I knew we would have to save money and life with a gambling addict means there are never any savings. Ever since we first started seeing each other Pete always said he wanted to take me to Barbados. So it meant the world to him that we were able to go there for our honeymoon.

Pete chose the area with the nicest beach and I chose the hotel. It was one he hadn't been to before, so it was extra special for us. We flew out there three days after the wedding, both exhausted after the culmination of such an emotional time. It felt like a fresh new start for us. We were finally married and had plans to set up our company. It was an exciting time. I knew I wouldn't go back to the NHS and planning this new business was an important achievement for us. All of Pete's adult life had been out of control and this was the opportunity for him to have control. He had gone from one extreme to the other, from being in a pit of despair to living a life free of addiction and running a company. Pete had wanted to get married for such a long time, but I knew we had to wait until he had conquered his demons. I was finally Mrs Shilton and he told me that he was the happiest he had been in his life.

I was in paradise. The resort was idyllic and when we got into the room I went straight on to the balcony. Staring at the tropical gardens and the beautiful beach and looking out at the Caribbean sea, I was so overwhelmed that I literally sobbed because I knew that the ultimate dream had come true. We had made it and had finally come through the other side. This was something that could never have happened whilst Pete was gambling, and this is why it was so precious to us.

We are fortunate to be in a position where we get invited to numerous celebrity events but we much prefer to attend and support charity functions, which we do often. We are far happier walking on the beach on Mersea Island or walking across the marshes with Charlie Buttons than posing on the red carpet. In fact, we are at our happiest and most comfortable in our wellies wandering around our lovely island home, then popping into The Coast Inn, a lovely pub overlooking the estuary where Pete can have a pint of his favourite Doom Bar and freshly made fish and chips. We had enjoyed holidays and happier moments even during Pete's time gambling, but there was always the dark cloud hanging over us. Now we are totally free. For Pete this life is better and happier than any kind of life he led before.

Along with the birth of Missy and the arrival of my grandchildren, Pete quitting was one of the greatest moments of my life. After everything we had been through I knew that, for Pete, this was the ultimate prize. Life after addiction is full of wins and full of dreams, however large or small.

CHAPTER 10

LIFE AFTER GAMBLING

PETE'S STORY

I am now in the best place in my life I have ever been. I am with Steph, and we are delightfully happy and still very much in love. I am free of gambling, thanks to Steph's help. We own our own home, a beautiful, large bungalow which we've worked really hard for over the last few years. We are close to the beach and can walk daily with our little poodle, Charlie Buttons. I feel so lucky.

I'm free of the burden of all those financial problems that dogged my life before and brought me to the point of depression and financial ruin. From 2006 to 2015 – the year I finally stopped gambling – I had lost a staggering £800,000!

I kept my football life separate from my gambling, but the double life I was leading was an enormous strain. To be free of it is a wonderful feeling. Yes, of course, I could be a lot richer, in terms of money in the bank, but I am richer so many other ways that aren't money here with Steph.

The best goalkeepers are the ones that make fewer mistakes, and I made fewer mistakes than most in my professional life on the pitch. Off the pitch, yes, I made a lot of mistakes. In my double life I made so many mistakes it was untrue and, at the root of all those mistakes, was the one big mistake which was my gambling. Yes, I've lost a lot of money and, in this book, I have confessed for the first time just how much I have lost to gambling and more to failed business ventures exasperated by those gambling losses. But I hope I've also shown that anyone similarly caught in the trap of gambling addiction should not feel guilty but should *do* something to ensure that they stop. You can put your past behind you, finish with gambling and start afresh.

Yes, money can make you happy, but only if you use it in the right way. I realise that this can appear to be a flippant thing to say in a world where many struggle to earn enough money. You don't have to have a lot of money in order to be happy. I know people living on the breadline who have a wonderful family, and they find happiness in so many ways. Equally I have met many multi-millionaires who, for lots of reasons, are far from happy despite their wealth. Of course, there will be some people on the breadline who might say "I don't know what I'm talking about" as they hardly have enough to pay their bills. Everyone is entitled to their view. I think the key is having control over your money and that is something that a gambling addiction robs from you. Money becomes something you need to find to feed – not yourself and your family – but your addiction. Addictive gamblers have to find the courage, find the trigger and the good reason to stop. It may well be that they finally realise the devastation they have caused for their loved ones or that they are causing to themselves. They need to find that inner strength and find those who can help them stop.

The goal is to find a better way and a better life. You will never get that big win through gambling, and what you do gain will be at the expense of other people, mostly those closest and most precious to you. Remind yourself that £5 in the bank is better than £5 on a horse or on the spin of a roulette wheel, because you will eventually lose that fiver for sure. Even if you do win, do you feel that compulsion to try again and again? If so, you will eventually lose. And that pleasure of a short-term win, turns into long term despair, desperation and depression.

I had Steph to make things hit home for me She was the main reason I stopped. You too can find that reason to stop. It might be to save your relationship with a partner, a parent, a child, a sibling or a dear friend. Or it might be to save yourself. You might have borrowed from friends and family to fuel your betting and you are desperate to pay them back. You won't repay that debt by continuing to bet. That must be faced and dealt with. There is no point digging a deeper and deeper hole. There is no win big enough to outweigh the win of kicking a gambling addiction.

So, here I am. I have not gambled in six years. I am still running my own company where I have regular and enjoyable work as an after-dinner and motivational speaker. I also have regular work as a pundit when England are involved in the big tournaments such as the European Championships or the World Cup. Thankfully, no one has forgotten what I achieved in my career – that I played in three World Cups – and it's still recognised that I have a lot to offer to the game. These days, every club has a goalkeeping coach and techniques have changed. Goalkeeping coaches from overseas have brought new ideas to the Premier League. Techniques have changed although, in my eyes, not for the better. I wanted my way of playing to be remembered and preserved. In 2019, my gambling days behind me, I made a film outlining the fourteen different techniques that I built my footballing career on and would recommend putting into training exercises for teams today. I called it *Shilton's Secrets*.

Steph and I make a reasonable amount of money and now, for a change, that goes straight into our bank account not to the bookmakers. I am lucky to have a healthy football pension, plus my state pension. All in all, it gives us enough for some of the luxuries in life such as lovely meals out and holidays. My main consideration is that Steph and myself are very happy. In fact, I've never been happier. If I had a million in the bank it wouldn't possibly make me any happier.

So many people judge happiness by the amount of money you possess, by the size of your properties, and how many cars you have parked in the underground car park of your mansion. It's especially true of how the public view footballers. Lots of people think that applies to former players particularly if they have reached the kind of status that I managed in my career. But it doesn't quite work that way. Top footballing salaries today are vastly out of proportion to whatever the biggest stars of my generation of professional football were paid. The game has become vastly more lucrative for players. It may well be true, on reflection, that footballers like myself were never really cut out to be businessmen. Perhaps I allowed myself to be taken advantage of. Sometimes it's easy to believe that people who become so wealthy had to step on people on their way up. I don't think that's true of me though. I hope I am remembered for what I achieved in football and with affection by my friends and my family. Looking back on my life, I am proud of it and hopefully I've left a football bootprint that will never be forgotten.

CHAPTER 11

GIVING HOPE TO OTHERS

PETE'S INSPIRATIONAL STORY

Here is something interesting to ponder on: as I became a committed punter spending so much time, energy and money on gambling I also naturally became a favoured client of the bookies. In fact, I became such a valued customer that, every Christmas, William Hill and Ladbrokes sent me a massive hamper to say thank you to me. I would also regularly receive invites to the races, with full on VIP privileges. All these gifts were obviously in the hope of keeping me gambling. At the time I was hooked on gambling and so just thought the gifts were great little bonuses. I've now come to realise that the companies were sending the gifts out to the losers or, as the gambling company would call them "the good customers". When that realisation hits you, like me, you may feel a bit deflated, used and taken for a mug. Of course, I now know that gambling is quite simply a mug's game. But that's impossible for you to see when you're stuck in the addiction.

The pleasure of a short-term win turned into long despair, desperation and depression but I still found it impossible to stop. Eventually I met Steph and things hit home for me. The fear of losing Steph and the realisation that, whilst I was gambling, I was not a winner but a loser – these were the things that turned me around. You too can find the reason to stop. You must believe you can do it. That belief cannot come from anywhere or anyone other than yourself. Stop, look and you will find it. Don't hide from the realisation of the truth, pull it out to the forefront of your mind. Think of the other things you could be spending your money on, rather than throwing it down the drain in the direction of the bookies. Think of holidays, cars and nice days out or even smaller things.

Something – anything – that will make you happy and content with your life that you couldn't possibly afford while you're gambling. Once you have quit, you could be saving for something special, paying back debts to friends or clearing your credit card balance. You could slowly come back into the black and not worry yourself sick watching your money disappear. Just those thoughts could be all the inspiration you need to have a reason to quit.

You could redirect your energies into some physical activity, even if it's simply walking or running, something to make yourself feel better. You don't necessarily have to start a fitness regime, but any form of physical activity is good for the body and also good for the soul and the mind. The point is to find *something* to do. You might rekindle an old interest or start a new one – anything to fill the space which used to be filled with gambling.

Gambling can rob you of your friends, alienate your family and leave you without a relationship which can lead to a feeling of emptiness. That emptiness only feeds the gambling, so it increases. Try forcing yourself back into relationships with friends and family. Look for people to support you in your recovery. Don't be afraid to reach out.

There are good counselling services available for people with gambling addiction. For me, that was never an option. There was no way I could have gone to a counsellor – I would never have felt comfortable divulging my perilous financial situation that I had hidden from the world for so long. Perhaps it was my own celebrity that made me feel this was never an option, but it is for others. Don't be afraid to go down that road and ask for professional help.

Like coming off any addiction there has to be a period of adjustment in your life. It's important to commit and leave that past behind. A cut off can't be half-hearted. You can't say "I'll stop for a while and see how it goes." An alcoholic's only salvation is to never take another drop of drink. A gambler's only salvation is that there can never be another bet – not even a few quid just for fun. If you do, you go straight back into addiction. Your addiction will try to make excuses that you are better off gambling. That there is no harm in just one last bet. This is false comfort. If you want to enrich your life the best way is to stop gambling. I can't reiterate enough, there's no point in an alcoholic saying he's giving up then after a few weeks treats himself to half a glass of wine thinking that will be OK. It's not. It leads to the full bottle, then another bottle. It's the same with a gambler. *Stop means stop*. It means forever. It means a new life.

Don't be afraid to cry out for help when you struggle. Trust me, you will need help from wherever you can get it. When you first decide to quit you don't think that new life is possible, but it is. Of course, you'll have withdrawal feelings and you'll be tempted to get back into the habit. Sadly, there are vast amounts of gambling opportunities for you, all urging you back. These times are, what I call, "trigger moments" – like a pop-up advert on social media or betting companies and horse racing adverts on TV. These trigger moments will try to entice you back into gambling and this is when you must be strong. Believe you are a winner. Find that inner strength. Do whatever you can. Reach out for help if you need it. Put tools in place for dealing with that trigger moment – go for a walk or anything that will take your mind off it and switch it off. These trigger moments will occur often when you first quit but, trust me, they become less and less frequent and last for less and less time. Once they start to decrease, I promise you, they eventually disappear completely.

I was extremely lucky because I have never had a relapse but I must address the subject of dealing with them. I'm no expert but it's clear that any addict can relapse during withdrawal after quitting. This problem can occur when one of the trigger moments come along and your tools aren't enough to fight it off and stop you being pulled back into addiction. Basically, the trigger and the bookmaker can have a winning moment. Whatever happens, you must not beat yourself up if you should relapse. Dust yourself off and get back up. As goalkeeper, if you make a mistake in a football match it can cost the game. The first thing you do in that position is dig deep inside yourself and see how that mistake happened so you can learn where you went wrong. Then in your next match you can come out fighting and knowing that you're not going to let that happen again. A goalkeeper sometimes lets a goal in, but you can't let your team down or *yourself* by giving up on the rest of the match. You must get back on your line, focus and do everything in your power not to let another one in. After a relapse get straight back into re-sharpening your tools. Remember your reason or reasons for quitting. Give yourself a reality check. Quitting might mean you repay your debts, mend your relationship or save for the thing that will make your life better. Try to remind yourself that, with gambling addiction, you are living in a false world. Revisit your tools, put them into place ready for when the next trigger moment comes and realise why yours haven't worked this time. You may need professional help and that's fine, just reach out for any tool that you think you need. Ultimately, when you make the life changing decision to stop gambling, you need to commit to the idea that *stop means stop*. You might have had a wobble on the road to being gambling free but please don't lose heart. Keep positive. You can do it. If, after 45 years of being a chronic gambler, I can quit then, trust me, anyone can.

You must realise gambling addiction is an illness and it's not your fault. If you earn a million pounds a month, you will lose a million pounds a month… a gambling addict will lose everything that's in their account and more. Eventually it catches up with you. Be under no illusions that top footballers or famous individuals can *afford* a gambling addiction. It makes no difference who you are, or how much you have – if you're addicted you will lose it all. That's the problem and that's exactly what happened to me. I was the game's top earner at the height of my football career. I had so much coming in that it allowed me to think I could afford to lose money because I could cover the losses. It took me 45 years to realise I was losing every penny I earned. I'm under no illusion that same thing would have happened if I'd been on a million pounds a year as today's footballers are. In fact, I think it's easier to get hooked nowadays because of smart phones and the freedom to gamble that the internet offers.

Take one day at a time. You may be only at the start of your journey overcoming gambling but it's the biggest start of your life. Maybe, like myself, a light suddenly comes on in your head and you see what gambling is doing to you and that you are really getting nothing positive in your life from it. You're just losing money. From that great "light coming on" moment of realisation, you have work to do. It's said that a lot of addiction recovery is best taken one day at a time. As with any illness, it takes time, so pace yourself. You and nobody else has made this decision and only you can finish the job off. People around you can help enormously but, ultimately, it's only you who can do it.

Gambling addiction is a mindset. It tells you that the only way you can win is through gambling but that's not true. On your path to recovery, you are winning. After time, you will need your tools less and less and your debts will become less and less. Remember to reward yourself during your recovery, congratulate yourself and be proud of what you've achieved. And remember this quote told to you by Peter Shilton who heard it from a top executive of a major gambling company: "Ninety-nine per cent of punters *lose*."

You can do it.

Pete.

CHAPTER 12

STEPH'S COSY SOFA CHAT

We moved into our forever home in 2019 and it managed to give us complete closure on our old life. In our new home we don't have the TV/gambling room anymore but just off our main lounge we have a small room that we've nicknamed Steph's Prosecco Lounge. It has a cosy, dusty pink sofa with cushions on it and it's here that I can sit with friends, family and Missy for coffee or – OK – the odd glass or two of bubbles! It's wonderful that I now feel comfortable that the ones I love can visit our home, relax and generally have a lovely time.

The old, relaxed Steph slowly returned while Pete was in withdrawal. It's strange – when I recently asked my closest friends if they were aware of any difference in behaviour in me when Pete was gambling they all said no. I obviously hid my double life as well as Pete did. I am possibly not alone in that behaviour and I should imagine quite a few partners of gambling addicts can relate to me.

I'm so lucky to have wonderful friends in my life who I think the world of and feel the same about me. When your partner is going through something like gambling addiction, even if you can't open up to them, just having them around in your life can be of great comfort and they can offer you a huge distraction from all your problems. This was certainly the case for me. My friends might not have known the full story, but they were still invaluable support for me.

It's been such therapy for me to be able to sit in my Prosecco Lounge with family and friends and freely talk about our experience. It is also great therapy as I sit here now on my pink sofa writing my words of comfort to you all. I want to speak from the heart to all the loved ones out there that may be feeling lost, alone or confused. I want to tell you that I understand entirely what you are going through.

It has been so emotional writing this book and looking back on those dark years of Pete's gambling days. They were memories I had buried. To be honest, from the moment Pete quit I just kept moving forward, never daring to look back for a second. Having a famous partner makes the situation slightly more difficult. They are even more used to living their lives discreetly. Pete is a well-known public figure who has come out and publicly told his story. I think that is incredibly brave of him – so admirable and selfless. I can't tell you how proud I am of him for doing this. I had sacrificed a lot to get Pete to where he is now. Despite working in the NHS for most of my adult life, I lost out on my pension, gave up the rest of my career and a large salary. But, ultimately, it was a small price to pay. I have absolutely no regrets as, deep down, I always believed he had the determination to win the battle inside him.

As a loved one or a friend of a gambling addict life can be so difficult. Certainly, if you live with the addict you also become a victim – the silent forgotten victim. For me it was doubly hard as Pete was such a beloved and famous figure. I remember a time, during those dark years, when I was trolled on social media and accused of being a gold digger because of the age difference between Pete and I. Trolls were accusing me of only being with him for his money, saying that he was a Sugar Daddy and once I was even accused of just waiting to receive his inheritance. That remark was so painful that it really reduced me to tears, as it couldn't have been further from the truth. All this just added to the hurt.

I've stated numerous times in this book that gambling addiction is an illness and a disease. This is a true "Steph quote" and one that I stand by. We must all keep those words linked together when we describe this awful addiction. And I am keen to speak to the loved ones who really are the forgotten and hidden victims. When the gambling world has got a grip on your friend or loved one it plays havoc with your emotional and mental well-being. I wish I could offer you a magic wand – a quick fix to help you overcome the problem but, sadly, I can't. However, I can offer you some of the tools that I used to help Pete and maybe some of them might work for you. I also hope I can offer you much comfort along your journey of helping your loved one through a gambling addiction.

I wonder what your perception of a gambler is. Can you picture what a gambler looks like? Now I can tell you from my experience that often gamblers are highly astute, some are professionals, hold down good jobs and often have loving families. They can also be dedicated, hard-working individuals. These kind of gambling addicts are hard to detect and they are the bookies' favourites – their best customers. This gambler will excel at work. The better the job they do, the harder they will work. The more they earn, the more they can gamble. But remember, some may not be able to work or are out of work. Imagine being in a room at a social event with me and there are several hundred people around us. Could you honestly stand with me and identify the gambling addicts in that room?

Let's start at the beginning, the moment when you may feel that there may be a problem. Perhaps you've seen signs or, like me, you may have a hunch, a gut feeling or an intuition that something is wrong. That may be all you have to go on, so please trust your inner voice as I did mine throughout the entire journey. You will then need to become the investigator, the financial stalker – and please don't feel bad about doing this. Remember, in order to help your loved ones, lines must be crossed, something that you would never normally do. I know it's uncomfortable but, seriously, it's part of the help and support you can give in cracking into the addict's world. It's not an easy thing to deal with. I wrestled with the idea of snooping into Pete's financial affairs but I eventually realised it was the only way forward. Incidentally, I never did manage to find or work out Pete's password for his betting account on the laptop!

So, how do you ascertain if your loved one has a problem? You should start with looking for the signs. Are they being secretive? Are they acting a bit shady? Are they starting to have moods swings? Are there ups and downs in their behaviour? They could be withdrawn. They might start losing relationships with friends or loved ones. Are they avoiding certain people or things? Are they being more reclusive than normal? Look out for and study patterns of behaviour and moods. Remember the highs and lows could be to do with the wins and losses.

If you are experiencing domestic abuse of any nature or have children or a family member being neglected because of a gambling addiction, my advice is to get out of the situation.

Parents who suspect their child is gambling must trust their instincts. Gambling addiction is the hardest to diagnose as there are few physical signs. Trust your inner voice. Teenagers in particular are often even better at hiding things than most adults and sadly some parents just don't know how to handle mental health problems. You must tackle it, deal with it, face it head on and with the right support and understanding the family can come through it. It's very difficult for parents because we are the enforcers of discipline. You have to remember you are dealing with an illness in your child so this will need to be treated with great care and understanding.

Once you are pretty sure there is a problem with your loved one's gambling remember you may have some big shocks coming so please prepare yourself. Detach the person from the addiction – really try to separate them in your mind and see the addiction as the disease. Like I did, be determined to try and wrestle your loved one back from the clutches of the gambling companies and beat the bookie.

As a loved one, in particular a parent, try not to blame or ask why the one you love has this illness – and you must see it as an illness. Trust me, trying to find a reason can tie you up in knots. Looking at Pete there could have been a whole host of reasons why he'd fallen into a gambling addiction. Could it be genetic? Did he become addicted to the buzz of a win during his career in football? Was he groomed, or enticed in by slick advertising? Was he just bored or lonely? Should the football industry have taught him lifestyle and financial management skills? Did he have mental health problems? It could have been any one of these or a culmination of all of them. Why does it even matter? What purpose does finding a reason give? Trust me, there isn't one. For Pete and I, it was about moving forward and definitely not looking back for a reason to blame. For me it served absolutely no purpose as it wouldn't change anything in the past.

As the partner of a gambling addict, it's helpful if you can protect yourself financially whilst you keep up the investigating. I know this isn't possible for everyone. I tried numerous times to get Pete to have a credit report done as this would have shown me the true extent of his financial history but at the height of his addiction I didn't stand a hope of persuading him to face the truth. When he quit we did submit to a credit report, knowing the reality of the situation really helped us both on going forward. When you are confronted with the extent of a loved one's problem – try not to look shocked and stay calm in front of them. Assure them this is a problem you can solve together.

Start openly talking about dreams for the future with them. Encourage trust and openness and try to let them know you're there and you will understand. Most of all be patient. It's hard at times not to feel hurt. The shocks can feel unbearable, and you will feel angry for all the anguish you're living with. But just keep thinking positively. I placed all my emotional grievance on the bookies and the industry and not Pete.

With help, support and people working together anything can be dealt with. But prepare yourself for the fact that it can be very hard. With mental health issues, drink or drug addiction, there are forms of help that you can get from the GP but sadly there is no course of medication – no magic pill – that can tackle gambling addiction. Keep being positive for the recovering addict. The most import thing is they have made the decision to quit and that, in itself, is the best start for a new and exciting life. I can't stress enough that I never put pressure on Pete. I knew his gambling addiction placed him under constant pressure and stress and my adding to this would have only driven him further into the addiction. Ultimatums, I felt, were totally unfair and there was a strong chance that they would have made him worse.

By gently threading the words "win" and "lose" into conversations you can start to tap through psychologically and start to change the addict's understanding of those words. You can make the suggestion that gambling companies are the only winners and pundits will always, ultimately, be the losers. Try replacing the word "win" with "lose" in some of the articles covering the betting industry to give evidence that it's the bookies who are winning.

Now, when Pete speaks in interviews and conversations about gambling or within the pages of this book he states that he was always losing. I think I must have brainwashed my poor husband because we still both use the word "lose" every time we talk about gambling. Maybe I'm proof that you can change an addict's mindset? You can change their belief that gambling means winning to realising that gambling means losing – in many aspects aside from the financial loss. I guess it's like learning a new song. You must keep practising the words, over and over again, for it to register in your mind and enable you to sing it.

As part of the road to recovery, all addicts will have debts to pay. Debt is one of the biggest symptoms of a gambling addiction. The recovery is long and can be difficult and the fear of them relapsing is great. Physical and mental withdrawal symptoms are one side of it but there's often a financial recovery and that may take years to clear. But remember, nowadays there is far more advice and support to help people work through and get out of debt. It's important to let the addict know this and help them find organisations that can assist in this side of the recovery.

The addict must find their own reason to quit. Sadly, you can't do that for them but, with time and understanding, you can get there. It's imperative that, after they quit, support and help is there. This is a crucial point in recovery from the illness. Don't tiptoe around the subject of gambling, gently bring it into regular conversation. Educate yourself, research as much as you can – knowledge is power. Look for signs, trust your gut and become the investigator. Protect your own finances, if you can, to mitigate the damage. Remember, money feeds this addiction just as alcohol feeds the alcoholic and drugs feed the drug addict – *they are no different to each other.*

I only found out about the true extent of Pete's losses in the summer of 2020. I can say now that I was absolutely devastated for him but obviously I didn't show it at the time. I placed my resentment and the blame at the feet of the gambling companies. Like me, when you find out the reality of how much one addict can lose, it will shock you, but you cannot show them that. When I saw the data on Pete's losses I needed time to process it. I ran a hot bath, shut myself in the bathroom and took some time out. I was genuinely heartbroken for Pete. This poor man had worked so hard –and, in a way, his hard work had served his country – and now he was left with nothing to show for it in terms of financial security. Pete had a strong legacy in football but any money he had earned from it had been pumped into the gambling companies during the years of addiction.

There will be a withdrawal process with any recovering addict. I would say it took Pete nearly three years to be completely free from the pull of the addiction. But then, he had been engulfed by it his entire adult life, so his recovery was bound to be far tougher and lengthier. Guilt must not be placed on the addict. The remorse they will feel is immense. The point where they decide to quit may be the point that they start opening up for the first time just as Pete did.

If you can reach out for support, it is out there for you. At the end of this book is an extensive list of organisations and charities you can contact for help with either your own or a loved one's struggle with gambling addiction. I now wish that I had looked for that support rather than battle through alone. Please, please don't feel ashamed for your loved one or for yourself. This is a condition like any other illness so don't let the thought of shame stop you asking for help. Reaching out is not a weakness – believe me, it is a strength. You may have insecurities about the addict in withdrawal having a relapse. For up to a year after Pete quit, I definitely had those fears. You will need time, patience and total understanding to help them through the withdrawal process until they get to the moment when they are finally free. If they do relapse don't be afraid to engage professional support. And don't give up.

I hope, with all my heart, that those of you trying to help a loved one with a gambling addiction can find some comfort in my words and maybe not feel quite so alone. I hope you felt welcomed into my cosy little lounge. And I hope I have reassured you that you can get through this. Don't give up. Be patient. Look for the light at the end of the tunnel.

With love, Steph x

CHAPTER 13

THE FINAL WHISTLE

PETER AND STEPH'S STORY: OUR RESEARCH

After Pete's recovery and what we had been through as a couple we wanted to explore how the gambling industry worked and how prevalent gambling addiction was. We knew we had to educate ourselves over the ethics of gambling. Within just twelve months, we learned so much. Sadly, the deeper we got into the subject the murkier it became.

Don't get us wrong – we know there are millions of people around the world who really enjoy a bet and gamble responsibly. It can bring joy, fun and excitement to so many. We have to make it clear that we aren't *anti*-gambling, however, we feel strongly that there must be safeguarding and protection in place for the vulnerable.

In early 2020, the CEO of a company that owns two of the gambling industry's brand giants and one of the most powerful men in the gambling industry gave evidence to a House of Lords select committee which was set up to look into the efforts to control problem gambling. He made a truly startling statement that shocked us both: "Ninety-nine per cent of the customers who play on our sites will lose." What an astonishing admission. It says it all. They want to make as much money as they can. At that same select committee hearing another gambling company CEO confirmed that there was a trend towards online gambling and that his company's strategy was to make this a priority. It is a greedy industry. In 2018 it was estimated that the UK gambling industry growth was worth £14.4 billion. It's become the Wild West out there.

We now all have internet access in our pockets on our phones. The convenience and ease of betting on your phone is a gambling company's perfect world – they had found their paradise. When the Covid 19 pandemic crisis hit the UK in March 2020, we predicted a dangerous time of growth for online gambling. One big betting company saw revenues leap by 106 per cent during 2020 mainly due to a significant rise in online gambling especially during lockdown periods. Lots of people don't understand how serious the problem is in the UK. In the past, the idea that someone could become addicted to gambling in the same way as a person becomes addicted to drugs was a highly controversial one. It was originally viewed as a compulsion not an addiction. Recent research now shows that gamblers and drug addicts have the same chemical changes in the brain that occur during their highs and lows. This justifies Steph's insistence that Pete's addiction and withdrawal process was identical to that of a drug addict. We already have an epidemic in gambling addiction. Sadly, unless changes come, this number will only grow. In a survey by Gamble Aware in 2020 it was estimated that nearly 1.4 million people in the UK were suffering with problematic gambling.

One of the reasons it will get worse is that there is a noted rise in children with gambling problems. In June 2019 the first gambling addiction clinic for children was opened. In October of that year experts reported that the number of children aged 11–17 with gambling addictions had quadrupled in just three years to 55,000. We have to question whether the gaming industry is really willing to bring in the safeguards necessary to avoid a whole new generation of children becoming hooked on gambling. We both feel we are on a crusade to make this happen and turn the tide of this gambling epidemic in the youth of today. One of the ways we can take action to help is to tell our story and that is how this book has come about.

We have dedicated our book to the memory of Pete's dad, Les, and to Missy, Steph's daughter. Les had always struggled with how to help his son overcome his addiction and the fact that he lived long enough to see Pete turn a corner meant everything to us. And it must have been so difficult for Missy, standing on the sidelines and watching our journey. She continues to support us 100 per cent and was one of the people who really encouraged us to write this book. She could see how many people we could reach and help. Her loyalty and love for us has been amazing – we truly appreciate it.

We also want to dedicate the book to Jack Ritchie and Lewis Keogh. Both of these lads tragically lost their precious lives to gambling addiction. We first read about Lewis in a newspaper article in 2017. A photo taken of a handsome, happy 34-year-old was accompanied by a report that stated he had taken his own life in 2013. Lewis was a footballer and club manager to Headingley AFC, had earned a degree in sports psychology from Teesside University in Middlesbrough and worked as a facilities manager. He had struggled with a gambling addiction that he kept almost entirely secret, even from his parents. Before he died, Lewis left a message for his parents and brothers explaining why he had to leave them. The last line read "Gambling is cruel, I need peace." The club and his parents still work to keep Lewis's story very much in the public domain. His parents, in particular, campaign in Northern Ireland on a quest for law changes in gambling regulations. They are truly inspirational. It was at that moment we knew Pete's voice could make such a huge difference and that lives needed to be saved.

Whilst researching, we came across the charity Gambling with Lives. We contacted them and Pete held a long telephone call with Charles Ritchie, the founder. He kindly spoke to Pete at length about the dreadful loss of their son, Jack. Jack's gambling addiction started when he was only 17 years old. At the age of eighteen his father became aware of the problem and took his son to every betting shop in their home town of Sheffield where they left a photograph of Jack and had him sign a form to prevent him placing bets there. Jack's gambling just moved online. His parents tried everything, even blocking his access to gambling sites but they were only able to do this for a year. Jack took his own life at the age of just 24. On the day of his death, he emailed his parents, Charles and Liz, to say that he had been gambling all day and felt that he could never be free of the addiction. Charles and Liz have been such an inspiration since coming out and telling their story. Their efforts to help other poor families who have lost a loved one to this awful illness is remarkable.

These brilliant, handsome young men, both in their prime, died because of gambling addiction. Both had adoring, loving families and both suffered such tragic, avoidable deaths. Along with the tragic stories of Lewis and Jack, in 2019 we began to notice more and more stories of people losing their lives because of gambling starting to appear in the press. We discovered the shocking statistic that there was a least one death a day due to this vile illness. We knew then that we couldn't sit back any longer. It had been almost six years since Pete had quit gambling and we both felt that, mentally and emotionally, he was now in the best place to cope with coming out and telling his story to the public. We knew we had to join in with others and try to save lives along with trying to support addicts and their loved ones. Steph felt that there was very little help and support around for the loved ones of addicts, so we really were compelled to help.

If our book, *Saved*, can change or save *just one life* then, for us, it will have been worth every second. In January 2020, we approached the *Daily Mail*'s business correspondent, Tom Witherow, who among other areas specialises in gambling stories and leads on their gambling campaigns, and also the producers of breakfast TV programme *Good Morning Britain*. We honestly thought that these would be one-off interviews. It wasn't at all easy for Pete – coming out and baring his soul to the world. He is still in demand globally and viewed as an international icon and he had never publicly discussed his addiction. Looking after his well-being was and has always been paramount to Steph. The coverage in the *Daily Mail* of our story was great. It supported our campaign to raise awareness accompanied by the story of our relationship. The morning that the article hit the shelves, we were in the *Good Morning Britain* studios to be interviewed by Susanna Reid and Piers Morgan. We did find that nerve-wracking. Pete was out of his football comfort zone and Steph prefers to stay far more behind the scenes in Pete's shadow. Steph was quite possibly the first footballer's wife to ever sit on breakfast news and tell the British public that gambling addiction was an illness and openly discuss the recovery her husband had made including his withdrawal symptoms. Steph's message was strong, loud and clear. Being interviewed by Piers Morgan can be very daunting for some guests. But, once she was on camera, Steph wasn't at all fazed. She dealt with it all brilliantly, knowing she and Pete had a clear message to deliver and Susanna, especially, seemed really interested in the story.

The response we received as a couple, from both the interviews was staggering – it was unbelievable. We received thousands of messages of support and love from fans. But, more importantly, there were messages from addicts, not just gambling addicts, who said they were going to quit because of Pete's story. We also heard from many loved ones whose partners were struggling – even some whose partners were in prison as a result of crime committed to fund their gambling addiction. These stories were heart rending. If it hadn't hit us before, it certainly did then – this problem was huge. It was massive. We felt totally overwhelmed. From then on, we knew we just couldn't walk away. We had to do more than just tell our story. We had to do more. We donated any fees from our interviews to Charles Ritchie's organisation, Gambling with Lives.

At the same time as undertaking the interviews, we had contacted Nigel Adams, the member of parliament for Selby and Ainsty who was also the current Sports Minister. We wanted to see if we could support future gambling awareness campaigns. We knew Pete would be a great influence and a huge voice for the cause. It was only a couple of weeks later that we arranged to meet Nigel at his parliamentary office in Westminster. Nigel has recognised problems in the industry, and he knew that these problems needed resolving. Nigel suggested we met with MP Carolyn Harris and Iain Duncan Smith who led the All-Party Parliamentary Group on Gambling-Related Harm. We met with them and both of us agreed to support the great work and campaigns they are doing.

We were then approached by the BBC's *One Show* to film a short documentary about our story. Again, this was hugely successful in raising awareness and thousands more messages followed. We were absolutely thrilled as, again, many were from addicts who were inspired to quit because of the film.

This was the first time we had spoken publicly about some of what we had experienced and the first time we really opened up so the show of support and the messages of hope we received were everything. It was at this time that Pete received texts from a few of the ex-England teammates he had played with and other people in the football industry. They wanted to show him their support.

Just a few months later in June 2020 the snooker legend, Willie Thorne passed away. We were good friends with Willie. Pete had worked on the after-dinner circuit with him for many years and we kept in regular contact with him. We were due to fly out to Spain around that time to support his charity golf week. We knew of Willie's struggle with gambling addiction. After Pete quit he reached out to Willie numerous times to try and help. Willie would always say; "I've just quit, Shilts!" When Willie passed away we were devastated. We were so fond of him. Willie's death felt like another loss in our lives that was entangled with gambling addiction.

Our aim now is to leave a legacy with our story, this book and our work with charities. We are both committed to supporting the All-Party Parliamentary Group on Gambling-Related Harm and feel strongly that the UK gambling commissioning regulators need an urgent review. The current regulations are not fit for purpose. It was formed, in 2007, originally to regulate and supervise gambling laws in the UK. Ironically, their stated mission was to "Keep gambling fair and safe for all." Throughout our entire journey we have not seen any evidence of protection for the vulnerable exercised at all. Where are the regulation laws that protect children against developing gambling addictions? Why are addicts are still losing jobs, homes, relationships and even their lives because of gambling? Where is the protection? Why are lawmakers not scrutinising gambling companies who are in breach of this duty of care?

We believe that there needs to be urgent action and a total overhaul of the industry. We feel strongly that gambling companies need to be held to account for the lives ruined and lost because of their product. If you were to get severe food poisoning in a restaurant that led to time off work and weeks of recuperating, you would be entitled to some form of compensation. Someone would be held accountable. But the gambling laws won't enable this, and so gambling companies have no accountability for the damage they cause. This was the hardest thing for us to learn: that those inside the gambling industry just don't seem to care about what has been destroyed.

The NHS and the government education departments also have a role to play. They should be offering a full education programme. Gambling addiction must be regarded as the same as drug or alcohol addiction as it has been proven to be. GPs and schoolteachers can be educated about this illness and taught to recognise the signs. There must be pathways in place to support people in recovery. These are things that we will campaign and push for until they are in place. If you think back to a world before the smoking regulations in 2007, the big tobacco companies advertised everywhere – like the gambling industry, much of the advertising used sport to add glamour and appeal. These companies, despite the health concerns surrounding smoking, were welcomed by the government because of the vast sums of taxes paid to the treasury. Eventually it led to a health crisis. First they increased the taxes on tobacco, then ordered that health warnings were placed on cigarette packets. Eventually advertising was banned, and public health stepped in with hard hitting campaigns. This process took *years*. We just hope the gambling companies will experience the same journey – only much faster because time is of the essence.

Saved has been, emotionally, very difficult for us to write but we pray it changes lives, educates and gives you hope. Above all else, we hope that by sharing our story it might *save* a life.

Pete and Steph

CHAPTER 14

POST-MATCH REFLECTION

PETE'S STORY

Whilst writing this book, Steph and I revisited our experience of living with gambling and, for the first time, we explored what it was really like from the other's perspective. When I quit, Steph vowed that we must never look back. We have just kept moving forward ever since so raking up the past has been extremely painful and, at some times, quite shocking. When you are a gambler you don't notice those you hurt. You really are totally unaware of how your behaviour affects your loved ones. You are emotionally detached and therefore fail to recognise any of their worry, hurt and stress. This is, of course, part of the illness. You are caught up in the world of gambling addiction and really blinded to anything else.

In this book Steph has spoken about her miscarriage for the first time. When I look back at that sad time I remember it being a very traumatic experience for us both. Despite our ages and even though we weren't trying for a baby, we still felt a loss. It would have been a much loved and wanted pregnancy. It was a very upsetting and painful experience for her. At the time, I felt so helpless and so upset for her. I can now see, having read her version of the story, why that was a fundamental moment in our relationship. It was the thought of any loss connected to Steph that was so significant in pulling me out of my addiction.

Steph is a spirited blonde with a heart of gold combined with a backbone of steel – she is not one to mess with! My nickname for her is Titch but, make no mistake, there is a giant within her. Steph's career in the NHS meant she was adept at providing loyal, unwavering support to people who are suffering. And her singing career, I think, gave her the courage plus the drive to be strong enough to stand by me despite the enormity of my problem. She also has a strong nurturing side to her which made her the perfect partner to care for someone in a state of despair. Steph's devotion to me shines through. Her kindness and love are inspirational.

I think Steph's been left with resentment towards the gambling industry heavily fuelled by her heartache at my experience of it. This emotion has festered ever since she first asked them for help. She was angry that they were unwilling to help and never held to account and she still wanted answers. Many people don't realise the recovery after gambling addiction doesn't end after the withdrawal symptoms stop. It can take years to clean up the mess caused. Steph was right, we did need to know where I had been let down. As does everyone who has been and still are being let down.

Where do the regulation laws sit when it comes to the gambling industry? To start with we knew that, legally, I was entitled to ask for my data held by Betfair regarding my betting account with them. I dealt exclusively with Betfair for nine years. They had made me – as they often do with heavy gamblers – a VIP customer, meaning I would receive all the inducements. I requested all my data through a data subject access request. By law, the company has to send you all your personal data concerning your account within one month of receiving the request. I requested mine on 11th March 2020. We made allowances for the fact that the Covid 19 crisis would undoubtedly affect response times but, having still not heard back from them in May 2020, we chased for it. We made several formal complaints to Betfair and on 6th August 2020 I raised the breach to the government's ICO departments (The Information Commissioner's Office). This office was set up to uphold information rights. Essentially they are the UK watchdog who enforce data protection laws. Unbelievably, I didn't hear anything from the ICO until 9th January 2021 – over five months later! The watchdog basically confirmed that the gambling company had not complied with data protection obligations, but the only action taken by them was a letter they were sending to Betfair reminding them of their obligations. The ICO never even checked if I had received my data, so it seemed to me that it was a waste of my time contacting them.

We finally received the data we requested from Betfair but not until September 2020 – six months after my request had been received. The data we received from the company was so complicated we needed it professionally investigated by an expert. Around this time, we reviewed Betfair's 2008 terms and conditions – which is basically what every new customer signs up to. They were 57,612 words long. Nearly as many as in this book.

The investigation results were emailed to Steph in a form of a report. I had an idea of my losses, but the report gave an in-depth analysis of my financial data held on my betting account. Steph did shed some tears as we learned the extent of my losses. Emotionally, it didn't touch me. I just feel I am out of the darkness of gambling addiction and that was a win. I beat the bookies because they can no longer hurt me but, for Steph, the emotion was very different.

The Gambling Act of 2005, which repealed the Betting, Gaming and Lotteries Act 1963, the Gaming Act 1968 and the Lotteries and Amusements Act 1976 was a huge improvement in many areas, but, like so many pieces of legislation, failed to keep step with the real experience of vulnerable gamblers like myself and the problems we face. In my opinion, it did not go far enough in proactively protecting gamblers, instead relying on 'customer-driven' actions such as setting limits on account deposits and cooling-off periods when what vulnerable gamblers need is active intervention from the gambling companies. As an example, if a gambler is going from stakes of £500 to £5 or less and then back to £500 stakes, then the betting companies should have an intervention triggered. My data clearly showed that on some bad days I would start with an £800 bet and then would end the day putting on small bets as low as £10. My betting history showed signs of irregular staking and gambling disorder traits. It was obvious I was a problematic gambler. The expert's report confirmed that I was a chronic addict. Betting companies should have a legal obligation imposed upon them to intervene where problematic, erratic gambling traits are evident.

After I decided to quit, Steph had secretly emailed Betfair pleading for help regarding my disorder. They had responded to her on 24th February 2013 by email and one piece of data showed that on one particular day I had placed £1,101.87 on bets and lost £637.92. If effective, proactive safe-guarding protections for vulnerable gamblers were in place, any betting company could have placed a temporary block on my account. Shockingly, what the data from Betfair also showed was that my losses totalled well over £800,000.

Even after I closed my account in 2015 they still didn't exclude me from their platform until 16th January 2020 – oddly just after we'd been interviewed on *Good Morning Britain*. It's difficult to think that I had worked so hard during my life and had lost nearly everything I'd earned to this awful illness. You have to realise that addicts don't just use their earnings to feed their addiction – they use finance and credit, credit cards and loans. I can't understand why, to protect especially younger people, credit checks aren't undertaken as they are when you open a bank or credit account. This way, surely it would protect the vulnerable as you could just have a set amount to gamble with.

After Steph sent the email to Betfair pleading for help for me, I went on to lose a further £52,000. In 2020, Steph wrote again to the company to ask for some form of refund as she felt I deserved it. You can imagine she got nowhere with that. At the same time, I wrote a formal letter to the CEO of Paddy Power and Betfair who was involved with a Premier League football club. I politely invited him to an online meeting with me and Steph to discuss our concerns. Astonishingly, he didn't even acknowledge my letter. It has since been reported by the *Irish Times* that this CEO's annual pay package nears 2 million Euros and includes a £622,000 bonus. I find it hard to understand how they can want to engage with football clubs yet not engage with England's most capped footballer and a globally known footballing figure at that. You would think they would embrace me as an asset with valuable real-life experience. I would make an ideal safeguarding ambassador if they are really trying to safeguard gamblers from addiction problems.

Stewart Kenny co-founded Paddy Power in 1988. In February 2021, he wrote a piece for the *Daily Mail* about the gambling industry and how to fix it. Here's what he had to say:

> *"When online gambling started to take off in the UK, I had been a bookmaker for close to three decades but despite my many years of experience, I failed to see the scale of the emerging challenge until too late.*

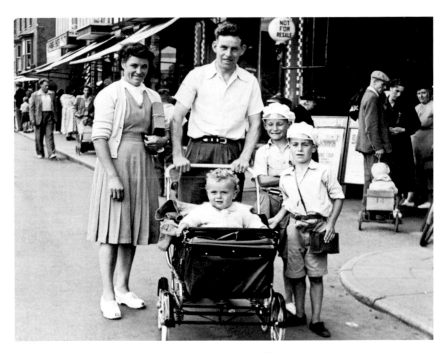

Picture Credit: Bob Thomas/Popperfoto/Getty Images

From our family album: on holiday in Mablethorpe with Mum and Dad
– that's me in the pram.

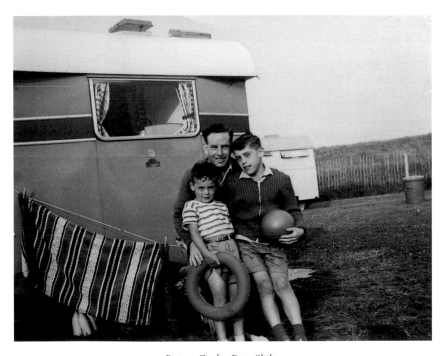

Picture Credit: Peter Shilton

Me, Dad and my younger brother by our caravan in Trusthorpe, holding my beloved
football – I'd wanted to be a professional player for as long as I could remember.

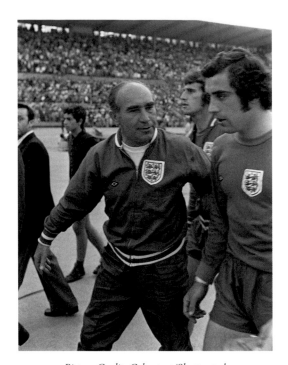

With my first and greatest ever England manager, Alf Ramsey after an Italy v England match, 14 June 1973 in Turin.

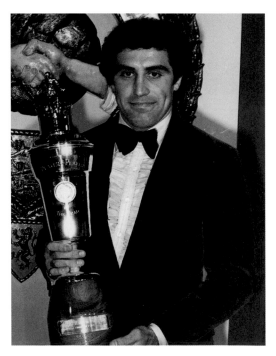

Receiving the award for PFA Player of the Year in 1978: to be given this prestigious award was a very proud moment for me.

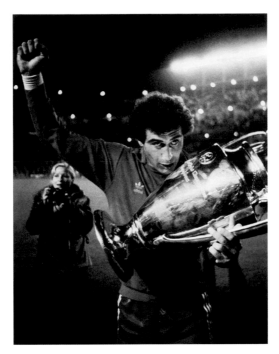

Picture Credit: Colorsport/Shutterstock

Celebrating with the trophy after Nottingham Forest won our second European Cup Final, beating Hamburg in Madrid, 28 May 1980.

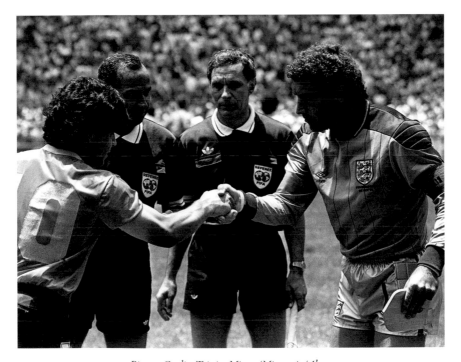

Picture Credit: Trinity Mirror/Mirrorpix/Alamy

The World Cup 1986 Quarter-Final – the infamous 'Hand of God' match – shaking hands with Diego Maradona before kick-off; the only time I ever shook hands with him.

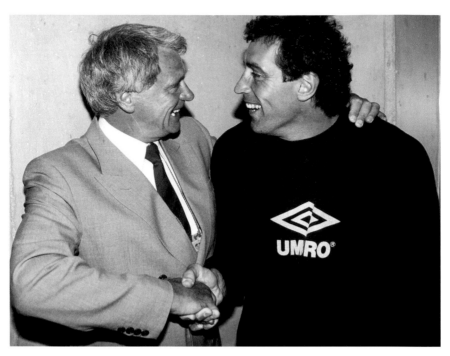

Picture Credit: Bob Thomas Sports Photography/Getty Images

England Manager Bobby Robson congratulating me after we'd qualified for the Italia 1990
World Cup. I made my 125th appearance for the country during the Finals.

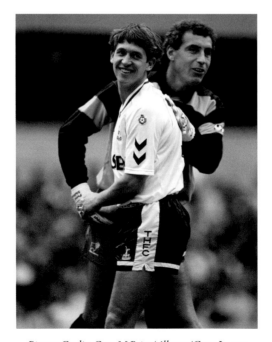

Picture Credit: Gary M Prior/Allsport/Getty Images

Having a laugh with Spurs' striker and England teammate, Gary Lineker during a League
Division One match between Tottenham and Derby County at White Hart Lane,
8 September 1990. We are still great friends to this day.

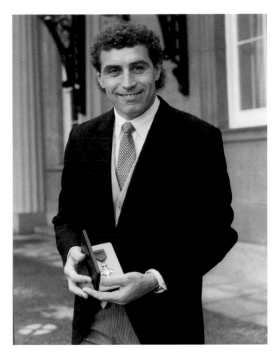

At the palace after receiving my OBE from Her Majesty The Queen.
It remains one of my greatest achievements.

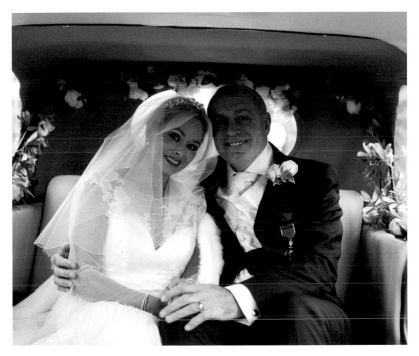

Our wedding day, 10 December 2016: fulfilling our dream with my Titch.

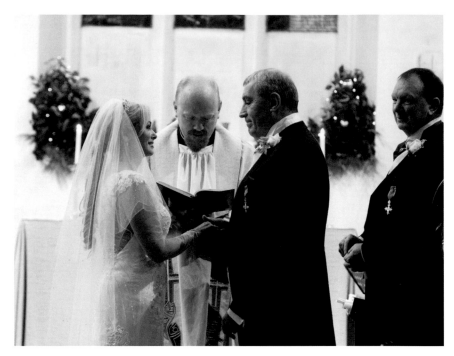

At the altar on our happiest day. Hidden in the service was our jubilation at my overcoming my chronic gambling addiction – we'd made it!

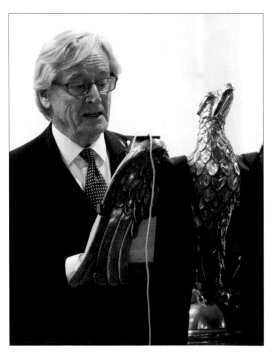

Bill Roache MBE reading Steph's wedding day poem at the service – I knew exactly what her words were saying to me.

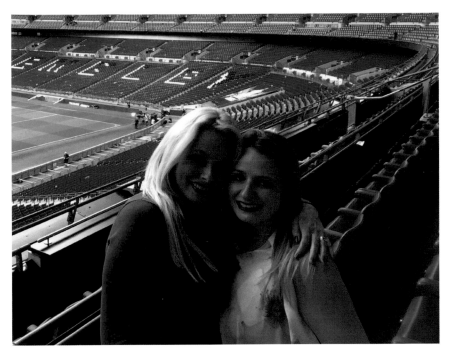

Steph and her daughter Missy (and now, proudly, my step-daughter) at Wembley
– my little rocks who have always stood by me.

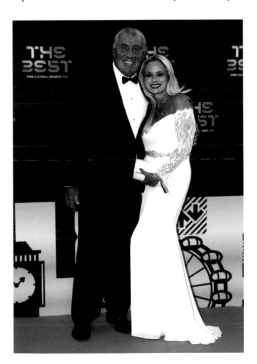

Now enjoying life gambling addiction free! On the green carpet with Steph before
The Best FIFA Football Awards at the Royal Festival Hall on 24 September 2018.

Picture Credit: Peter Shilton

Steph and me with Australian goalkeeper Mark Schwarzer, England Manager
Gareth Southgate and FIFA Vice-President David Gill at the Football Awards.

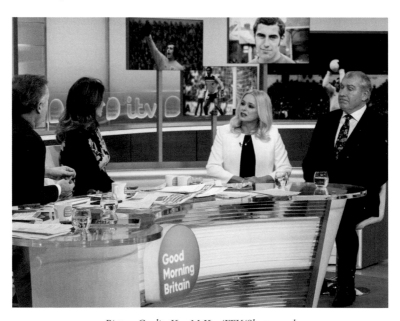

Picture Credit: Ken McKay/ITV/Shutterstock

Appearing on *Good Morning Britain* in January 2020 with Piers Morgan and
Susanna Reid. It was the first time I had ever publicly spoken about my 45-year
gambling addiction.

"I resigned from the board of Paddy Power in 2016 because of my concern that bookmakers were failing to take effective action to curb gambling addiction. In my view the industry was, and still is, doing not nearly enough to curb the addictive nature of some of their products.

"I regret to have to admit the excesses of online gambling have harmed thousands of families across Britain and Ireland but, despite the compelling evidence, the industry unfortunately remains in denial. The gambling companies may have to sacrifice some of their profits – maybe up to 15% – in order to make some products less addictive and the government needs to drive this.

"I acknowledge that I shoulder some of the blame for the harm caused by the addictive nature of some online gambling products. I wish I'd been a lot more proactive. The fact I did not do more leaves me with deep regret."

In my opinion Betfair and Paddy Power treated me and Steph with total disregard. I think Steph is right, during my 45-year chronic addiction the gambling companies and the regulations hugely let me down. And they are continuing to let down millions of others today.

JON HOLMES' (Pete's first football agent) STORY

Peter Shilton was my first big-time client. I've been privileged and lucky enough to work with some of Britain's most successful sportsmen: Gary Lineker, David Gower, Mike Atherton, Will Carling, John Barnes and Ruby Walsh. All of them possessed special talents and reached great heights of accomplishment but, amongst them, nobody showed more single-mindedness, professionalism and dedication in their quest to excel – to become the best in the world at their chosen discipline – than Peter. Comparisons are hard to make with different eras, codes and visibilities but some stand out. My late friend, Hugh McIlvanney, arguably the greatest sportswriter in the English language wrote that Peter "was almost certainly the best goalkeeper living." For me he will always be that.

Coming from Leicester, I had always been aware of Peter. He was dubbed England's finest ever schoolboy international goalkeeper. I remember standing next to his goal when Leicester Boys lost out to Chester-le-Street in 1965 on the Saffron Lane home ground. The following year, the team, Peter and two others from the team would find fame. Alongside Peter, Jeff Blockley, the Coventry, Arsenal and Leicester centre-back, and Romeo Challenger, who became Leicester rock and roll band Showaddywaddy's drummer, became English schoolboy trophy winners.

I followed Peter's progress with the England boys' team, signing first for Leicester City and later making his England full international debut. When I first began my career as an agent he was my number one target client. We met up, discovered common ambitions and ideas and started a twenty-five-year business and personal relationship.

Together we negotiated transfers, endorsements, media engagements and the creation of the image of a footballing superhero – a super fit world star. It was rewarding and fun and brought financial rewards and, in our own fields, fame and respect.

But there is always a backstory, the reality behind the image and the media spotlight. What made Peter so successful in his sporting life, was a single-minded obsession with developing his craft symptomatic of an addictive personality. I knew he followed the horses and liked a bet; addiction lay there as well. One day, early on in our relationship, we took a trip to Leicester races. In receipt of a tip, we placed our bet. I won £40 and was ecstatic. This was 1973 and well-paid footballers earned £100 a week. I was earning £40. Peter pocketed over a thousand pounds but seemed strangely indifferent. How much had he staked? I was well aware not all tips proved correct. Bookmakers don't lose money. Peter was always secretive about such matters. And so a pattern emerged. However many deals we did, however lucrative the new contract, Peter was always wanting more. He was always short of cash, had always "had a bad run lately" and so his cash flow was "a bit tight".

The success on the field that followed his transfer to Forest didn't seem to offer any respite. More money led to bigger bets, bigger wins but bigger losses. On one occasion, in 1979, Peter rang me to say he had won the tote jackpot that weekend of £25,000. He wanted to make some proper investments. He did. On horses. A week later there remained nothing left to invest in anything reliable.

At one point I called Brian Clough, with whom I did not get on with, desperate to enlist his help with dealing what had clearly become an addiction. Peter had returned from a gambling and drink fuelled bender at the Cheltenham National Hunt Festival, many pounds poorer. There were always those happy to hang around in his company, basking in his celebrity glow, but unwilling to help him confront his issues. Clough, in my opinion, was never in awe of Peter's ability as a goalkeeper, in the way that Peter Taylor, Clough's assistant, a former keeper himself, was. Clough's driving force was his desire to control people and mould them to his ambitions and plans. He saw Peter as fundamental to his team, so was keen to maintain that control. I may be a little unfair, but I saw no attempt by Clough to tackle Peter's addiction. But, by bailing him out financially from time to time with contract amendments, he retained control over what he saw as a prize asset. Did he care about Peter as a person? I don't know, but once the problems got out of control, Peter was moved on to Southampton and the pattern continued to Derby and beyond.

On one occasion, Peter went behind my back to a good friend and business acquaintance of mine to get a loan. I realised that he had lost touch with reality and the addiction was eating away at his morality. On another occasion just a few weeks before Italia '90, the Derby manager, Arthur Cox, rang me concerned that Peter was being pursued by bookmakers about unpaid debts. Both Arthur Cox and his manager at Southampton, Lawrie McMenemy, were aware of the problems, and tried to help, but the addiction was too strong. How anyone could continue to play at the top level whilst wrestling with this? One can only marvel at the mental strength it must have taken and yet also despair at the level of addiction that gave rise to such misery. Extraordinarily, despite the financial chaos and the domestic problems that inevitably follow from such circumstances, Peter's playing standards never lapsed. He was England's number one and undisputed as the world's best. It is a testament to his ability, dedication and addictive (in a good way) personality.

I remember games throughout his career where he showed incredible brilliance. There was the European Cup Final against Hamburg, when he withstood all that Kevin Keegan and co. could throw at him. I remember Jimmy Greenhoff, thumping his fists in the mud in despair as Peter saved a succession of seemingly certain goals. There was his debut for Stoke at Wolves; out of the world saves against Scotland at Wembley; a display against Queens Park Rangers that rained superlatives from the doyen of football journalists, Brian Glanville; and wonder saves at Coventry as his team won the First Division title for Forest.

Watching a game at Forest with the late Keith Weller, a fan engaged Keith in conversation, "He's a great keeper," he said of Phil Parkes, Rangers' international keeper. "He's a very good keeper. But the guy at the other end (Peter) is a brick wall," responded Keith.

Eventually Pete and I gave up on our business relationship. I felt that I had failed both him and me. I had argued with him on countless occasions, even lied to conceal some of his money to prevent it pouring down the bottomless chasm. We never really fell out, but I couldn't get through. In an autobiography, Peter later spoke about turning down an attempt to tackle the problem that I had devised with Arthur Cox. "Why I turned the offer down, I shall never know. Jon got fed up and went off to work with Gary Lineker. They have been very successful and deserve it." Peter was still punting at the time of writing that – a generous and wise spirit laid low by gambling, and that addictive nature.

I still retain the greatest respect for Peter, as a player and as a person, more so now when I hear that, with Steffi's help, he has confronted his demons. He continues to need our support and will always do so. Addictions and an addictive personality are lethally destructive forces.

There's just one last memory I would like to share in conclusion. A couple of years ago, myself, Peter and Peter Schmeichel were in conversation in the Leicester boardroom after a game. "You two are the greatest keepers it has ever been my privilege to see," I said, "but Shilton you were the best." Schmeichel never said a word.

PETE'S STORY

People have asked me numerous times why there seems to be a high number of gambling addicts in the football industry. I have to say, straight away, that a majority don't turn to gambling. However, the character instincts that make a professional footballer and the determination to win, are ideal credentials which could lead on to problems with gambling. Most successful professional footballers have instincts such as an addictive nature, never wanting to give up, needing to live on a high – all fertile ground for gambling addiction. These, along with the long periods of boredom players experience between the high points of training and playing – all potentially open the door to gambling.

It's interesting to note that Jon Holmes felt that friends latched on to me in the early days. Plenty, during my gambling years, did take advantage of me. Sadly, this is a hazard of being a professional footballer, everyone's always wanting something from you. You can't really trust anyone and people can use you. It can be a lonely existence, both during and long after your career has finished.

I was lucky enough to have Jon as my business manager/agent at a time when it wasn't fashionable in the '60s and '70s. I met him while I was playing at Leicester City. We soon formed a good, solid relationship – one we both also found financially rewarding. He always knew I liked a bet but in those days, I thought it was under control. It did eventually become a problem between us. Jon talked to me, advised me that I should stop but I always thought I knew best. I regret the path I took. After we split I realised that I could have been in a far better position if I had listened to Jon. I was so strong-minded, which was a big positive for my football career, but not for my gambling addiction. When I eventually stopped and overcame my illness I could see the mistakes in my past off the pitch much clearer.

I am so pleased Jon kindly agreed to be part of this book. His input is very much appreciated as is the resumption of our friendship – proving it's never too late to make amends. Most importantly, though, I'll always be grateful to Jon because there was one thing I did take his advice on and that was putting large sums of money annually into a football pension which secured me for life.

If you go back to my prologue at the start of this book you'll remember how my first experience as a child of gambling was when my dad had that big win. You'll also have read in Gary's kind acknowledgement what an impression I made on him when he used to attend football matches with his dad. For millions of football fans in the UK the love of the game comes from fantastic childhood memories. Children are shaped by their earliest experiences. I am living proof that gambling *does* have an impact on a child. I truly believe that gambling does not belong on a football pitch It is morally wrong to have betting companies advertising at matches attended by families with young, impressionable children. Over the past few years gambling companies have encroached more and more into the world of football – glamorising gambling within the sport.

When Carolyn Harris MP kindly wrote her acknowledgement she stated, "We know how many football clubs rely heavily on the gambling industry for their income, especially in these times of great hardship for the lower league clubs. Many teams are suffering the devastating effects of the Covid 19 pandemic which has robbed them of the lifeblood of their industry – the paying customers. We can even take one of the biggest clubs in the world as an example – Manchester United. They have a global fan base. If a child is a Manchester United fan and they see a betting company on the front of their shirts they will associate gambling with their club. If they are loyal to their club, which a supporter will be, then that loyalty transfers itself to that betting company."

Gambling companies often offer highly lucrative endorsements to famous players. José Mourinho and Peter Crouch are two classic examples – both very high-profile men in the football industry, both very impressionable to football fans including children. I'm certain that if they knew the dark side of gambling they would possibly think again and not put their names to it. I have been told that gambling companies have sometimes outbid other companies by up to five times for a sponsorship contract at a football club. They almost have a monopoly. It is illegal to advertise gambling companies to children so how did this loophole happen?

In January 2021, Steph and I launched a campaign against gambling companies advertising on football shirts. I felt strongly that someone in the football arena needed to stand up and speak out: so the Shilton's Shirt Gambling Ban campaign started. We joined forces with The Big Step petition, a campaign created by a recovering gambling addict and Ritchie's Gambling with Lives organisation. One of my first campaign tweets on Twitter was read by 2.7 million people, with 190,000 people interacting with it. I believe that there are many out there that feel as strongly as I do – it's time for change.

I'm now personally in the strongest position I have ever been in to help others and to campaign with Steph by my side. I was out shopping with Steph a couple of years ago and we happened to walk past a high street bookmaker. The sight of it really gave me a nauseous feeling. This experience has repeated whenever I see a bookmaker's shop. I know it's because my mind and body realise what a place like that represents and what harm it can bring. Despite the obvious scars left from my addiction, I know I have truly won my battle against gambling and the bookies. Meeting Steph really was the turning point in my life. My dad called her a little gem and she sure is.

I want to leave you now, my friends, with this quote: "Addiction is giving up everything for one thing. Recovery is giving up one thing for everything."

Peter Shilton, OBE

STEPH'S STORY

When we're not in a national lockdown, often on a Sunday morning the front door opens in our bungalow and in pile my beloved grandchildren, Summer, Mollie and Louie, who I am so lucky to share with Pete, followed by Missy and our son-in-law, Dean. Missy always heads to the kitchen where I'm often found preparing a big roast. The children and our dog, Charlie Buttons, head to their toy room and gradually toys start to disperse and soon cover any floor space they can find. Dean heads straight to the lounge with Pete, ready for an afternoon of sport on TV and a couple of beers. Sometimes, when I take the boys in some beers, Pete will look up at me and our eyes will lock. As he smiles, I know he's saying: "I'm so happy." That relaxed, happy smile, along with a twinkle in his eyes was never there before he quit. The strained, weary face I once saw has completely gone. He's now at peace in his life and within himself. I can't tell you how wonderful it is to look at him every day and see happiness and relaxation written on his face. Isn't it amazing how a promise can be so powerful? I owe Pete's dad,

Les, a debt of gratitude for giving me the strength to be able to deliver on my promise to him.

I'm so privileged to share a life with Pete. I am truly grateful every day. It's an absolute honour to have been able to help him overcome his gambling addiction. I will leave you now with this thought – it's ironic how one of the greatest goalkeepers in the world, himself, needed to be *saved*.

EXTRA TIME

PETE'S CAREER STORY

One of the proudest moments for myself and my dad was when I signed apprentice forms for Leicester City at the age of fifteen. I was paid the princely sum of eight pounds per week to play for the club for the duration of a two-year apprenticeship. I'd turned down similar offers from the mighty Manchester United and Arsenal because it was my dream to stay at Filbert Street. The pay was the standard rate for apprentices, but my dad had been offered all sorts of other inducements by the bigger clubs who wanted to sign me. He never told me until much later and even then never told me exactly what the offers involved, but you can imagine – clubs are happy to throw money around when they wanted to sign a player. But my dad did things the right way. He wasn't a rich man, but he turned down the big clubs because he felt it was the right thing to do for me. "It's best for you," my dad told me. He was right.

When I was a kid, football was the all-consuming part of my life. It wasn't that I wanted to be rich or famous as a footballer – it was all about the game. I look at the money that's in the game today and I have to laugh. None of the football players I knew back then (even World Cup winners like Gordon Banks) were millionaires. I just wanted to be out there in the park or in the street, kicking a ball, diving to make saves, stopping shots – being a goalkeeper. Back then, nobody wanted to be in goal, but that was the position I always wanted so I always seemed to be able to find a few lads to have a game. Nobody ever had to persuade me into being the goalkeeper. I was more than happy being between the sticks. From the age of seven I considered myself a goalkeeper. That's all I dreamed about. I was simply football mad. From a young age, I was totally committed to working hard, training hard and practising hard toward my ambition to be a professional footballer.

Around the age of about ten or eleven, I found wasn't growing as fast as I wanted to – goalkeepers needed to be tall. I did try playing a few other positions, midfield, or striker – but I still did stretching exercises on the wall in my bedroom and anything else I could to make myself bigger. Then I had a growth spurt and I was back in goal as quickly as I could.

When I got picked for Leicester under-11s, I started to think, "I must be quite good at this." It is hard to imagine but, back in those days, the club training academies didn't exist. Clubs would scout schools and colleagues and you played in the hope of someone spotting you. I was at Court Crescent primary school which, along with all the primary schools in the Leicester area, would send a couple of their most promising players for an assessment at the club's training ground every year. You had a proficiency test on your skills – heading, dribbling and goalkeeping – watched by the club's coaches and some of the players. If you passed, you got a certificate.

Two of the coaches at Filbert Street, Burt Johnson, the club's first team coach, and George Dewis, a former club centre-forward, who turned out to be my mentor, invited me to train with the semi-professionals and amateurs each Tuesday and Thursday. I wasn't old enough and wasn't supposed to, but they saw something in me. They said I should turn up an hour or so before the others for my session. I cannot tell you how thrilled I was at the invitation. I would get on my bike after school to make my way to the football ground as quickly as I could, change in the teams changing rooms, – which was something special – and then do an hour or an hour and a half with George before the proper training session started for the older boys and men.

We are now very familiar with the state-of-the-art training facilities enjoyed by today's top teams, where no expense is spared, every luxury is laid on and the vast array of pitches look like billiard tables. But this is as far away from top flight football back then as you can imagine. The training took place in the Filbert Street car park. Fortunately, it wasn't concrete, it was more like shale surface. But it certainly toughens you up at a very early age. I was also playing with older boys than myself. Maybe that is a problem these days – some of the kids have it far too easy in an academy environment and that could be why so many fail to make the cut into the professional game.

As I progressed into the Leicester under-15s, my big ambition was to play for England Schoolboys at Wembley. First, though, I had to be picked. My team did remarkably well in the Schoolboys' FA Cup, and we played Swansea Boys in the final. The first leg was at a packed Vetch Field with a 12,000 capacity crowd watching and we drew 1–1. The second leg was played in front of more than 20,000 fans at Filbert Street where we again drew 1–1. We shared the trophy. Those matches got me noticed and I got a trial with England Schoolboys. I had a great game in the second trial match and got picked. So, there I was playing in front of 90,000 at Wembley for England. We beat Scotland 3–0.

Matt Giles was manager of Leicester City when I signed as an apprentice for the club and he was fully aware that I was much in demand by the big clubs. He told my dad, "Don't worry, when Pete is seventeen and he can sign as a professional player, we will look after him." And he was true to his word. That was typical of Matt, he was a tremendous manager, but also a man you could trust. Although bigger, more glamorous clubs wanted to sign me, I wanted to remain at my boyhood club, the club I had supported as a kid and the club who had nurtured me as a player.

It was anything but "glamorous" being an apprentice footballer back in those days, and that would be the same whether it was at Old Trafford, Highbury or Filbert Street. I signed on as an apprentice with about five other boys, and we were all paid the same and all treated in the same way. There was no preferential treatment and that applied even if you made the breakthrough into the first team. Our jobs, after training in the mornings with the rest of the players, were to wash the kit, clean the boots, polish the boots, wash down the dirty baths and clean the dressing room floor. Even in the summer, during the off-season, we had to paint parts of the ground.

I was in the youth team for around three or four months before I was promoted to the reserves. It was quite a leap for a fifteen-year-old. Much later in my career, when I was at Nottingham Forest where Brian Clough and Peter Taylor were in charge, Peter told me that he had watched me play in the Leicester City youth team. Peter was a renowned talent scout and he told me how he kept an eye on me in particular. He had a special interest because he had been a goalkeeper himself but, until he told me, I had no idea I'd caught his attention that young.

I was still an apprentice when I made my debut for Leicester City. But it wasn't the life changing call up to the first team – far from it. They didn't postpone the league games to make way for international matches in those days and Gordon Banks was away playing for England. I had already been elevated to the reserves which was quite a feat for someone so young. Making the leap into the first team so unexpectedly made no difference to my lifestyle. I was still earning eight pounds a week and I still had to do all my chores. I remember that match so well. It was an evening game against Everton and, after a warm-up session with the first team that morning, I still had to do all my apprenticeship jobs. I even put my own kit out in the dressing room ready for the match in the evening when all the other first team players had left. At 2 p.m. I was allowed home to prepare for the match where I had a sleep and a bit of tea – probably something like scrambled eggs. Then I reported for the match with all the other first team players. I had a good first game against Everton and we won 3–0. At sixteen, I had just become the youngest to play for Leicester City.

That didn't give me an excuse to slip out of my apprenticeship jobs the next day though. I was in the ground the next morning at 8 a.m., cleaning all the first team boots and the dressing room. Put it this way, I wasn't spoiled when I made my debut! Looking back, this was, a great lesson for me. It helped me to keep my feet on the floor and be level-headed. It taught me that the game was a tough profession and nothing would come my way without hard work, determination and total commitment. You wonder whether the current generation are taught similar attributes, but I doubt it – certainly not to the degree we had to endure. I kept a clean sheet on debut and went on to play 339 games for the Foxes.

As a boyhood fan, I grew up watching City play at Filbert Street, inspired by the man I would go on to replace between the sticks for both Leicester and England, Gordon Banks. People ask me what I admired about Gordon, and the main thing for me was his positional play. He always seemed to be in the right position before a shot was hit. I played four times for the Leicester City first team before my seventeenth birthday when I could turn professional. I was able to play those games because Gordon was away with England. There were still other clubs interested in signing me. Leicester City took the long-term view and decided to sell Gordon Banks to Stoke City as I had already proved I was ready and able to play in the first team. With Gordon off to Stoke, I instantly became a first team regular with a lot of pressure on me. Gordon wasn't just one of my heroes, he was a World Cup winning goalkeeper.

During my first year, in October 1967, I even managed to get on the scoresheet during a match away at Southampton. My long kick was lost in the mist and eventually ended up in the back of the net to make it 5–1. Incredibly, I was unaware I had even scored for a few moments.

I didn't learn until much later, that Brian Clough and Peter Taylor, who were at Derby County at this time, tried to buy me at this time. Brian Clough rang the Leicester City chairman, Len Shipman, who was also President of the Football League at that time. Len was a wily old fox – a fitting chairman of the Foxes! The club had a history of being open to selling their best players from time to time to balance their books and Cloughie knew that Leicester was suffering a bit of a financial wobble at the time. Cloughie offered Len £200,000 for me – which was an awful lot of money in those days. Len said that he felt that was a reasonable offer and one that he thought he should take to the board, for consideration by the directors. "OK, put the offer in writing, Brian," he told Cloughie. Brian Clough duly sent Len Shipman a formal offer to sign me. Instead of approaching the directors, Len took the written offer to the club's bankers who, once they saw me as so much collateral, opted to agree to an earlier request from the club to increase their overdraft. Shipman went back to Clough to inform him the club had turned down the offer as they had now solved their financial problems. Of course, Len never did tell Cloughie how he used his offer for me to get the terms he wanted from the bank.

I was perfectly content at Leicester and delighted when we reached the 1969 FA Cup Final. The FA Cup has become less important to teams these days. But, back then, it was one of the most important trophies in world football. The event was broadcast with a huge build-up live on TV.

We had beaten Liverpool in a memorable fifth round tie after a replay at Anfield. We had drawn 0–0 in the first tie at Filbert Street and were given little chance of progressing. But I saved a first-half penalty in front of the Kop, before Andy Lochhead scored late on which sealed victory and a place in the quarter-finals. Another 1-0 win, this time over West Brom at Hillsborough, got us into the final at Wembley. Leicester City had been to the FA Cup Final three times before and we desperately wanted to win it this time. But we lost by the same score line to Manchester City after Neil Young scored early. The FA Cup was the only trophy that eluded me during the whole of my career.

Unfortunately, as a team, we had taken our eyes off the ball once we reached the final. We had a players' pool, every team in the final did, and there was a lot of commercial stuff going on round the team. We were relegated to the Second Division at the end of that season. Frank O'Farrell stayed as our manager and we bounced back in the 1970/71 season, winning the Second Division title. In 1974, we come close to the FA Cup Final again, reaching the semi-final, before being knocked out by Liverpool, with the Reds getting their revenge for that fifth-round defeat five years earlier.

In November 1974, I followed in the footsteps of my predecessor Gordon Banks when I signed for Stoke City for £325,000 which was a world record fee for a goalkeeper back then. I could have signed for Derby County, and there wasn't much between the two when I came to make up my mind about which club to join. Brian Clough and Peter Taylor had left Derby and Dave Mackay had succeeded them in controversial circumstances, but that wasn't the reason I went for Stoke City. One of the reasons was that the Derby pitch was a quagmire at that time. The only bits of grass ended about two yards the other side of the white lines. I felt it would be very difficult for a goalkeeper playing week in and week out on a mud heap of a pitch, trying to dive around a goal area that was in such a poor state. Another was that Stoke's manager, Tony Waddington, had such a great reputation, I felt it would be a good move to play for him. And, of course, Gordon Banks was also associated with the club, although by this time he had finished his England career and had retired from playing football.

ENGLAND – HOW IT ALL STARTED

During my career, I played at every single level for my country: England schoolboys, England youth (now under-18s), the under-23s (now under-21s) and then the full England team. I think Terry Venables is the only other player who has done so too.

I was still playing Second Division football with Leicester City when I was called up for the under-23 tour behind the Iron Curtain where we played against East Germany, Poland and Russia. The day after I returned home from that, I got a phone call telling me that I was being promoted to the full England squad. Gordon Banks's father had died, leaving only Gordon West as a goalkeeper on the squad. So I went to Mexico, to join the tour that was designed as preparation for the 1970 World Cup Finals.

I had to quickly pack my bags and rush off to the airport. The FA fast-tracked my travel visa and I just about made the flight. There were two games scheduled against Mexico. Then matches against Uruguay and Brazil. Gordon West played in the Azteca against Mexico in the first game of that tour. But Gordon had to unexpectedly fly home. So, I played in the second game against Mexico. It was at another stadium and was called a B International so didn't count as a full England international match. So I was still waiting to earn my first cap. But playing with the Charlton brothers, Bobby Moore and other members of the '66 World Cup winning squad in that game was something very special for me. Gordon Banks flew back to Mexico to play the matches against Uruguay and Brazil. I was on the bench in the Maracanã where Pelé played in front of a crowd of 200,000. Even from there it was such a great experience.

Sir Alf Ramsey picked me to join the 28-man squad for the Mexico 1970 World Cup. At that time, England was blessed with so many world class keepers, and Alf went with Gordon Banks, Peter Bonetti and Alex Stepney. I had a month out there training with some great players and goalkeepers. It was a great experience because the ball moved a lot quicker through the air at that altitude and, as a goalkeeper, you had to make adjustments to your game to deal with that. You had to move a split second earlier because of the speed of the ball. The pitches in Mexico were also very dry and hard so you had to adjust to play with a ball that bounced a lot higher.

Alf Ramsey was the best England manager I played under and very similar to Brian Clough in his management skills. He had total respect from the players. He had such confidence but without being arrogant. He didn't burden the players with a lot of unnecessary chat, so when he said something, you listened. When we arrived in Mexico he didn't want the players sunbathing. We were only allowed to go in the sun when we were training, so you can imagine there were a lot of card schools in the shade going on, but not heavy gambling, but more to pass the time. After a week, this became monotonous, so the players had a chat amongst themselves, and decided to send a delegation consisting of Bobby Moore, Bobby Charlton and Geoff Hurst to see if they could change Sir Alf's mind about sunbathing. Sir Alf – or Alf as the players called him then – agreed we could have ten minutes on our front as a squad, and when our trainer Harold Shepherdson blew his whistle we could have ten minutes on our backs. When Harold Shepherdson blew his whistle again, we had to go back into the shade. Not really ideal or what the players wanted. But it's a sign of the sort of ship he ran that under his watchful eye the players carried out this bizarre sunbathing routine.

One day, Alf had to go in and speak to the England doctor, and wasn't there to supervise us during our brief spell of sunbathing. Quickly, the players decided to rebel. When Harold Shepherdson blew the final whistle to indicate it was time for us to move into the shade, nobody moved! Harold pleaded, "Come on, lads, you must go in." He blew his whistle again but still no one moved again. "I'm going to fetch Alf out if no one moves," he declared. After blowing his whistle three more times with no action he decided to fetch Alf. When he returned a minute later with Alf, everybody was in the shade. Nobody was going to cross Alf Ramsey. Alf Ramsey commanded respect.

Being in the squad was such an eye-opener for me. I learned from the top players like Bobby Moore, Bobby Charlton, Geoff Hurst, Martin Peters and Alan Ball behaved in terms of handling the pressures leading up to a World Cup. And I also had the experience of training with three great goalkeepers, including my childhood heroes, Gordon Banks and Peter Bonetti. I had always admired Gordon for his playing style. I admired Peter because, being on the small side, he was so agile. His nickname was The Cat.

I was disappointed not to make the final 22, but I had expected it. I always knew Sir Alf was going to play his most experienced goalkeepers. I was out there to cover for any injuries as well as to gain experience. We were given the option to stay or go home, but four of us – myself, Brian Kidd, Bob McNab and Ralph Coates – opted to go home. Peter Thomson and David Sadler decided to stay on. I felt like I would be a spare part, just hanging around. I watched the games at home of course. And it was in disbelief that I watched as we lost in the quarter-finals to Germany having been 2–0 up. Peter Bonetti deputised for Gordon Banks, who had taken ill, during that match. Peter was blamed for the loss later but, in my eyes, I thought he was unfairly treated. England lost that infamous quarter-final 3–2.

I made my debut in November 1970 against East Germany whilst Alf rested Gordon Banks. For me, it was such an honour to play my first full international. It really is every schoolboy's dream and it meant that I had now played my country at all levels. The game went well for me and I made some really good saves. In an echo of my fluke goal for Leicester City, the first thing I did in the match was to kick a long ball out of my hands down to almost three quarters the length of the pitch. Allan Clarke flicked the ball on for Francis Lee who ran through and scored. I suppose it was quite strange to see a goalkeeper making his first action almost making an assist on his debut! Martin Peters and Allan Clarke added to that goal scoring from a Bobby Moore deflection for us to win 3–1.

After that game I was elevated to the number two goalkeeper, behind Gordon Banks, for the next couple of years. When Gordon Banks was tragically involved in a car accident in October 1972, I took over as number one for England. I felt very sorry for Gordon and, obviously,

I had wanted to prove myself worthy of the place, so this was not the ideal way for this to happen. I got my chance to prove myself though. One match that allowed me to do that more than any other game was a game against Scotland at Wembley in the 1973 Home International Championships.

In those days most of the players in UK football were Brits – mainly English or Scots – so the rivalry between the two national teams was intense. If you lost against the Scots, you spent the entire year until the next game hearing about it. With ten minutes of play to go, Billy Bremner took a corner which we cleared to the edge of the box. Here, Kenny Dalglish struck a sweetly hit volley flashing into the top corner to my left. I went for it with my left arm but realised I wasn't going to make it. Instinct took over and, using my right, I managed to fingertip it away round the post. Even now I get Scots coming up to talk to me about that save in a begrudging, yet nice, way. That clean sheet against the Scottish team is one of the great memories of my career.

October 1973 also saw one of my worst memories in one of the most infamous matches in recent times for England as we faced Poland at Wembley. We needed a victory to qualify for the World Cup the following year. I watched the vast majority of the action from the opposite end of the pitch where Jan Tomaszewski, was making headlines with a string of outstanding and sometimes lucky saves. Midway through the second half, a slip by the late Norman Hunter allowed a Polish breakaway allowing Jan Domarski to score. If you're playing for England and let a goal in, especially in such an important tie, *everybody* remembers. Domarski hit a fierce shot from just outside the box which came straight at me. I was in two minds, wondering whether to stop it with my hands or my legs, but the pace of the ball beat me. A swift equaliser from a penalty by Allan Clarke was not enough. We drew the match and didn't make the finals. Does anyone ever ask me about the five or six saves I later made when we played Poland in a match that helped get us to Italia '90 and then into the semi-finals? No. I still get asked about *that* goal from 1973 though. You get used to it.

It still fills me with huge regret that we didn't qualify that year. At the time, I told myself I had plenty of World Cups to come, and I would end indeed up playing in four. But it was a massive blow missing out. I thought long and hard about that goal and my technique changed as a result. I changed my starting position: bending my knees more, getting down lower and a lot quicker. The next game was against Italy which we lost 1–0 with Fabio Capello scoring the winner. He later went on to manage England!

Sir Alf was sacked in May 1974. I was shocked and, to a degree, I am still shocked he was sacked. He was a great, great manager. Bobby Moore was also coming toward the end of his illustrious England career. Bobby was not only a football icon, he was also a really nice fella. He had the unique ability to be a great leader as well as one of the boys, which is not easy to pull off. Players had a lot of respect for Bobby, not only as a player, but also as a captain. I always got on very well with him and got involved with him on one or two projects off the pitch after he had finished playing. To win the World Cup on our own soil was what dreams are made of. It was sad that the man who had managed England's sole World Cup triumph and the man who led out that iconic winning team, should end their careers effectively on the back of that horrendous night against Poland. Both Bobby and Sir Alf will always be legends of our game. Don Revie, an ex-Leeds United player, replaced Sir Alf.

I had started playing for Stoke City and I thought I made an impression in my first game at Molineux where we had drawn 2–2 only after a last-minute penalty. After that match, I caught sight of manager Tony Waddington as I walked past the board room. He smiled at me, a look that said, "Well done, Peter." He needed that performance from me after paying out such a massive fee. We were top of the First Division (now known as the Premier League) with capacity crowds of 30,000 attending each game and with some terrific talent on the team in the form of Alan Hudson, Jimmy Greenhoff, John Mahoney, Mike Pejic, Terry Conroy and Dennis Smith. But a glut of injuries was our undoing and we finished fifth at the end of my first season.

We had a slowish start to the next season and made halfway up the league. Then one night we had a horrendous storm. Stoke's stands were wooden and the storm tore the roof off one of them at the Victoria

Road Ground. The club weren't insured and they couldn't afford to replace it. The only way the club could rebuild was to sell some players to pay for it. Soon after selling most of our best players, we were fighting relegation.

To make matters worse for me personally, Don Revie seemed to firmly prefer my old friend, the late Ray Clemence, to me in his England squad. I got a call from Jimmy Greenhoff, who had been sold to Manchester United. He told me that Tommy Docherty, his manager, was keen to take me to Old Trafford. A week later, The Doc was sacked. This was quite a low point in my career, and I had to summon a lot of my inner strength and resolve to keep my spirits up. I needed a lift and wanted to speak to someone in the game whose opinion I respected. I decided to contact Brian Clough who was at Nottingham Forest at the time. I'd never met Cloughie but I knew that he had tried to sign me a few times in the past. I was a bit down and urgently needed lifting when I turned to him for advice.

Cloughie told me to meet him at a guest house behind Trent Bridge that he and the players used all the time. He and I got on like a house on fire. I told him how much I respected him and that I would respect and value his opinions about what I was going through at that time. We talked football for some time. It was just great to have a conversation about the game with someone like Cloughie. I revealed my main worry and that was that Revie said to me that there was nothing much to choose between myself and Ray Clemence. Yet he never seemed to give me a chance and it was just so frustrating. I told Cloughie that I didn't like Revie and that I didn't trust him. I didn't realise at the time that Cloughie also didn't like Revie, and that the feeling was mutual. I did sense, at the tme, that there was some ill feeling between Clough and Revie just by Cloughie's reaction to my statement. He just sort of smiled at me when I confessed my dislike for the new England manager.

That chat gave me a massive boost. Cloughie simply advised me to concentrate on my game, to not let anything else distract or worry me and to continue what I was doing – my best – and the rest would take care of itself. As far as the England team was concerned, I should just be patient.

In later years, I've often tried to think back on why Don Revie had it in for me. There are a couple of things that come to mind. Don came from Leicester. I used to write a column in the local paper, and I once penned an article praising his Leeds team, but I also criticised some of the tactics of his players. I said that they were prone to keeping the ball in a fashion that it was taking the mickey. When they beat Southampton 7–1, I described their play as unprofessional and unethical – in fact, I described them as "dirty cheats". Word got back to me that Revie took exception to my comments. I can imagine that didn't help our relationship get off to a good start.

On Sunday afternoon, when the England squad was gathered for training, Revie insisted that we all watch the second half of a Stoke game I had played the day before on TV. I knew the reason he did this was because I had made a rare mistake in that game. I had raced out and clattered into the Newcastle's forward, leaving the striker with the easy task of rolling the ball into the net. Obviously, the players gave me some friendly stick about it, which was OK. But when I turned round, I caught sight of Revie and was shocked. He was laughing and sarcastically applauding my mistake! He had just wanted to make sure everyone saw my mistake.

This was the lowest point of my entire career. Revie rarely gave me a chance to play on the England squad. Maybe he really didn't see any difference between myself and Ray and it was personal. Either way, I was out of the reckoning for the best part of two years aside from a couple of games. You'll understand when I say that I was not a bit disappointed when he quit the FA and headed off for a pot of gold to the Middle East. Despite being a great club manager with Leeds, his England career was a massive disappointment.

CLOUGHIE – A ONE OFF

When I joined Nottingham Forest under Brian Clough and Peter Taylor, I immediately noticed how the atmosphere at the club was different to any I had experienced before. It was plain to see that players worked together as one and everyone was relaxed and professional. I could immediately tell that the management team were responsible because they were in complete control and so well respected. Training was not at all complicated and every one of the players gave each session their all. Everyone knew what was expected from them and team spirit was good.

The team had won promotion to the First Division the previous year and, despite some cynicism from the press and the pundits, we went on to win the division that season. From my first game with them where we beat Aston Villa, with a 2–0 win at home, it was a dream come true for me.

Cloughie was a character. I remember that I attended a meeting with my two agents to discuss the move with him and Peter in his office in September 1977. We were told to go into a room and wait for a few minutes. About an hour later we were summoned to his office: "Mr Clough is ready to see you now." I'd gotten to know Cloughie quite well, so I wasn't sure why we had been kept waiting for so long. I was unsure what was going on, so I made sure my agents went in first as I followed. I was shocked to watch them both go sprawling across the room with papers flying everywhere. Cloughie was laughing from behind the door where he had hidden to trip them up with his squash racket.

The meeting didn't appear to go very well from there on. As we discussed the terms of the move to Forest, Clough had an air of seemingly being totally disinterested, at times staring at the ceiling and beating the racquet on his leg. After a couple of hours, and not making much progress, he announced, "Well, this has got us nowhere, hasn't it? And I'd prefer to be *somewhere* rather than nowhere. So, good day, gentlemen. Thank you for coming." Then he stood up, turned to Peter Taylor and said, "I'm going for a bloody meal." I was devastated. I really wanted to play for Clough and Taylor.

The next morning at 8 a.m., I got a phone call from Cloughie asking me to meet him and Peter at a local hotel. He wanted me to come on my own. As I walked into the room at the hotel, I saw an open bottle of champagne in an ice bucket and Clough and Taylor sat there. Within fifteen minutes I had agreed a good contract and had signed for Forest. We raised a toast.

As well as being one of the most charismatic managers of all time Brian Clough's eccentricity bore no bounds. His man management was both bizarre and brilliant but, more importantly, it was hugely successful. His whole ethos was team building. No prima donna behaviour was allowed under any circumstances. He simply wouldn't tolerate it. "All for one and one for all, and if you're not prepared to do that, on yer bike," was one of his famous sayings.

Clough and Taylor rarely turned up for training but, when they did, you would sit up and take notice. It is hard to imagine now but, at the time Forest didn't have a training ground. We used a nearby park. Our usual routine was to run from our city ground along the River Trent to the local park. Tall nettles grew alongside the area of the park that we used as our training pitch. The ground we trained on was awful – fit only for dog walking which took place regularly even as we trained. I remember one day when a man was walking his dog and Cloughie was yelling at him to "get off our training pitch." The surprised man scampered off with his dog even though he was perfectly entitled to be walking there.

At one training session just after we had gone to the top of the league, Clough and Taylor come to preside over proceedings. We had just started our warm-up when Cloughie shouted, "Right, run through those weeds and nettles and run around that tree and back." I'm sure he knew there would be moaning and groaning so he added, "Off you bloody go." It stung like hell, but I understood he was making a point. He expected his players to run through anything for him in a game, so in training he would expect them to run through a few stinging nettles. I think he did it because of our recent success. It was a way of him reminding us to keep our feet on the ground and not let it go to our heads. No other manager would have done that back then. And certainly not now when our pampered professionals are so used to their state-of-the-art training facilities.

Cloughie definitely had a unique approach to preparing for a game. In my first season at Forest, we got to a League Cup Final at Wembley. I missed, along with Archie Gemmell, as we were cup tied, but we did travel with the squad down to Wembley. Chris Woods played in goal. The final ended in a draw and the replay was set to take place at Old Trafford.

Cloughie regularly used to take his players off to a hotel to forge team bonding, and this time he took us to Scarborough for a couple of days before the replay match. He also liked nothing more than taking his players for a stroll – even in the middle of winter. He would call them "leg stretchers". Often, before games, he would lead us out on a walk around whatever city we were playing in. Cloughie insisted that, as players, we shouldn't be sheltered in our hotel and we should also see some of the sights of the city hosting us. The day before the replay, led by Cloughie, we set off along the promenade for a brisk walk to get some sea air. Cloughie spotted a pub, took us in and told us to order a beer or two. On the walk back, he suddenly stopped and ordered us to take off our shoes and socks and go for a paddle in the sea. "But it's freezing," you could hear the lads muttering under their breath, "we are going to catch pneumonia!" – all out of ear shot of the boss. Despite all the moaning, we inched our way into the freezing water. After a short period, we started larking around, splashing each other, laughing and joking. Yes, it surprisingly turned out to be great fun and a laugh. It released a lot of the tension in the build-up to the big game. When we came out of the water, of course, there were no towels, so we all had to put our socks and shoes back on to our soaking wet and freezing feet. But Cloughie was far from finished. He spotted a fish stand, selling all sorts of weird and wonderful shellfish, and he told us all to order whatever we'd like. And he also told us to make sure we said hello to anyone who came over for a chat or for an autograph. Can you imagine modern-day managers and coaches with all their analyst teams and nutritionists allowing the players to eat all sorts of unsupervised shellfish before a cup final, or *any* game? No, of course not.

It sounds bizarre and it felt so at the time we were doing it. Some of the players must've thought their manager was crazy. But when I look back, I can see what Cloughie was up to. We were about to head into cup final replay and he wanted to remind us who was boss, that what he said goes and that he understood how to win trophies. He wanted to keep his players feet on the floor – or in this case on the floor of the seabed – and to take the lads minds off the game.

Another team walk, this time through the streets of Amsterdam before our European Cup semi-final leg, was one to remember. We were quickly confronted by a group of Ajax fans who wanted to give us some stick. The sensible thing would have been to ignore it and stride on.

Not Cloughie. He marched over with great intent and gave them an ear bashing for being so impolite and rude. He pointed out that they were letting down their city particularly as, when their supporters came to Nottingham, they had been treated with the utmost curtesy. The fans apologised.

We strolled on, enjoying the sights of Amsterdam. Suddenly, we found ourselves in the red-light district, arriving at what can only be described as some sort of a brothel or a strip joint, or both. There were two massive bouncers outside. Peter Taylor seemed to start negotiating a block booking deal. We didn't go in of course, but we were crying our eyes out with laughter. Peter was a funny man.

Later on, Cloughie stopped at a bar and told us we were allowed two bottles of beer each. It wasn't long before we were having a great laugh. Eventually, Martin O'Neill observed that it was half past ten and all the Ajax players would be tucked up in bed by now.

"Aye," said Cloughie, "but none of them will be getting any sleep!" He knew that the opposition would likely be worrying about the game. In contrast, we were now totally relaxed. We went on to get the result we needed to reach the European Cup Final. Clough's preparations might seem unorthodox, but he was always looking for ways to relax the players. This ensured that his teams were perfectly ready for big games.

When the first £1 million footballer, Trevor Francis, arrived at Forest, he got a shock and a bit of a reality check. On his first day, he found he had no alternative but to use the rather rough club soap and towels, the same soap and towels we *all* used during our showers after training. On his second day Trevor brought in his own lovely scented soap and fluffy white towels. Cloughie was not impressed. He wanted all his players to muck in, and if that meant handling sub-standard provisions, then everyone was in the same boat. Poor Trevor had no idea that simply bringing in his own toiletries would cause such a stink with his new manager. I think it would be unusual for any other manager to have made an issue about this, but Cloughie certainly gave Trevor a hard time over it.

Cloughie's philosophy was an "all for one and one for all" approach and, to be fair, it did create a wonderful harmony and a togetherness. The team were a unit which I am sure fostered the environment that led us to winning so many trophies. We won the league in my first season which enabled us to enter the European Cup the next season. After knocking Liverpool, who had won the cup the year before, out in the first round we won our first European Cup by beating Malmo in Munich, 1–0 with a great header from Trevor Francis. The next season we reached the League Cup Final again and this time I managed to get my winner's medal when we beat Southampton 3–2.

The cream on the cake was getting to the European Cup Final again at the Bernabéu stadium in Madrid where we took on Kevin Keegan's Hamburg. It was "King Kev"'s last game for the German champions before moving to Southampton, and they were by far the clear favourites. As part of our meticulous preparations, Cloughie and Peter Taylor took us to their favourite watering hole in the Mallorcan resort of Cala Millor. After a light training session, I needed to practice some proper goalkeeping techniques. But there was no grass whatsoever – the sun had baked the surface and it was rock hard and hardly conducive to throwing myself around on the ground! I couldn't do my normal training which was important to me preparing for such a big game. One day we found a bit of grass and I started to do a bit of diving but the manager of the hotel whose lawn it was quickly came out and told us to clear off. Obviously, I was getting frustrated and so I had a word with Peter Taylor, who had been a goalkeeper once himself. He told me we would have a couple of days when we got to Madrid where we would have a lush grass pitch to train on. "You can have a couple of good sessions then."

When we arrived in Madrid, we got on the team bus to travel to our training ground. I was looking forward to a good work-out. But when we pulled up I saw, to my horror, that the training pitch was like a hard tennis court. There was no way I would dive on that as I might injure myself before the final. I was complaining again to Peter when Cloughie came over and asked what the problem was. I told him. Cloughie wasn't having any of it. "Well, you had better go and find some bloody grass, hadn't you?" he told me with that usual Cloughie tone. So, trainer Jimmy Gordon and myself did exactly as Cloughie said. Jimmy threw a bag of balls over his shoulder and the two of us set off in search of some grass.

Because we were in the mountains, the only bit of grass we could find was a traffic island about fifteen yards in diameter, with two trees on it! We put a couple of jumpers down – like jumpers for goalposts – and Jimmy fired shots at me. The drivers of the cars going around us must have been laughing their heads off. I managed to do two ten-minute training sessions – all the time with cars driving around us and hooting their horns. They must have been wondering who was mad enough to be doing that.

We had had a long season, 75 games, and we didn't have a big squad like the top clubs do these days. Trevor Francis was out with an Achilles injury and we were definitely the underdogs. The final was a back-to-the-wall display of defending with one moment of brilliance by John Robertson, our left winger, as he scored with our only shot of the game to give us a 1–0 victory. When people ask me what my personal highlights were while I was at Forest, this was one of them. I made four or five saves that I was very pleased with. It was a fantastic achievement to win the European Cup in two consecutive years. And I couldn't help wondering, after my unusual preparation in the middle of the traffic island, if I'd wasted all that hard training over the years. Did I really need it?

Another of my favourite Cloughie stories occurred before another of our European Cup Finals. This time we were playing against Malmo. We were sitting around in the foyer waiting for the team bus to take us to the stadium. Peter Taylor was entertaining us by telling some funny stories – relaxing us and taking our minds off the game. Our centre-forward Garry Birtles was one of the last to come down to join us in the foyer. He had deliberately left a bit of stubble on his chin whilst shaving. Clough was not amused when he spotted that. Cloughie wanted his entire team to be immaculately turned out with neat haircuts, smart club suits and ties – the works. He wanted us looking the part of professionals, and we did, as we knew he would be inspecting us. Beards? They were out. That's why he didn't not take too kindly to Garry's little stubble. Clough looked at him sternly and spoke to him even more sternly.

"What's that on your face?"

"Just a bit of stubble," Garry replied. "It's there to bring me a bit of luck, maybe to get me a goal!"

Cloughie stared at him. Clearly he was not impressed by the answer.

"We are leaving here in five minutes," Cloughie told him, "if you don't shave it off, you're not playing. Get it off."

Garry hotfooted it back to his room. I don't think I've ever seen him run so fast. A few minutes later he rejoined us, minus the stubble. But he had shaved in such a hurry that he now also had a few bits of tissue paper soaking up the blood where he had cut himself a few times with his razor.

Another game that I have great memories of with Forest was the day we won the First Division in my first season. The match was away against Coventry. Although we still had three games to go after that match, we just needed a point to win the league. I made a save during that game which is still replayed often on TV and social media. It was a point-blank header from their centre forward, Mick Ferguson, when I was on my near-post. The ball was hooked across the goal and, as I moved across, Ferguson made a bullet header from four yards out. I managed to instinctively react and pushed the ball over the bar. I wasn't sure myself how I did it, but I remember Ferguson sinking to his knees. He couldn't believe it hadn't gone in. Goalkeepers are usually remembered for when things go wrong, and when they make mistakes, but that save, and my England save against Scotland are still replayed today. I was pleased to make two or three other saves during that match which got us to a goalless draw. We won the league that day and it was another special moment in my career.

The season we won the league I also won the PFA Player of the Year trophy. It's unusual for that trophy to be awarded to a goalkeeper so it was a great honour for me and a fine end to what was a memorable season.

WORLD CUPS

When Don Revie left, Ron Greenwood, the old West Ham United manager took over as the England team. Ron was known for his strategy of playing progressive football. He loved *good* football. He also installed Don Howe as his assistant, who was at Arsenal at the time. Ron was a real footballing man and Don Howe added that bit of steel and expert at defensive play and set plays, and they complemented each other. I thought they made a really good partnership.

Ron Greenwood came up with the idea of me and Ray Clemence playing alternate games in goal. Ray and myself were good friends as well as rivals, but it wasn't ideal for either of us really. Any international goalkeeper wants to establish himself as the number one choice, but I suppose it kept both of us on a competitive edge. It also kept us both playing international football.

Brian Clough was still my manager at the time, and I recall he said Ron should make his mind up – and pick Peter Shilton. He felt that Ron Greenwood was indecisive. Typical of Cloughie, he always felt I was the best. But to be fair to Ron Greenwood, he assured myself and Ray that he would pick just one of us to play for the whole tournament of the World Cup in Spain in '82 – if injury or a really bad game didn't force a choice it could be either one of us.

After a year of alternating games, the World Cup loomed. We were told that Ron would announce which one of us would play in the tournament at a training session. You can imagine the tension that morning. Normally, Ray and myself would go into a corner and do some warm-up and goalkeeping practice together, but on this day I went to the left, Ray went to the right and we both sat waiting for Ron Greenwood to appear.

Ron Greenwood appeared, after what seemed like ages, but was actually just five minutes. Both Ray and I were pretty nervous but for me it was excruciating, as this would be my first World Cup. I'd waited eight years after we'd failed to qualify in '74. Ron started walking and then turned right towards Ray. I watched Ron put his arm around his shoulder and saw Ray's head drop. I suddenly realised he was telling Ray that he was going to pick *me* for the World Cup squad. Of course, I was overjoyed, but obviously I felt for Ray. He was a close friend and we had such enormous respect for each other. It was amazing to have two goalkeepers to select from for the World Cup team, but amazing also that we shared such a good friendship. Later, when we arrived back at the hotel we were staying at during training, Ray, as he always did, said nothing. We just carried on like normal. I always respect Ray for behaving so graciously, because he must have been gutted.

We flew, as a squad, to Spain for the tournament. The first three games were in Bilbao, a city in the Basque region. At the time there was a real terrorist threat from a group of Basque separatists and we were accompanied from the airport to the hotel by two security men with pistols who sat at the back of the coach. Ron Greenwood had told us we had a lovely hotel near the beach, but he had forgotten to tell us that we were going to have an armed guard. When we got to the hotel there were two more guards with automatic rifles awaiting our arrival. To make it even worse, when we got to the training ground for our first session, we found there was a tank outside. It made us all a bit nervous to start with. But, after a few days, the tank disappeared and things relaxed a bit more. But the guards remained during our entire stay.

We played the first game in our group against France and. I remember that it was so hot in the stadium with not a breath of fresh air. It was one of the hottest places I've played in and that includes Mexico. It was so hot that the individual numbers on our players shorts which had been ironed on, all started to peel and fall off. We won 3–1 with Bryan Robson scoring the fastest World Cup goal after 27 seconds. What a great start to our World Cup campaign. We then beat Czechoslovakia in a comfortable enough game. Surprisingly, we struggled to beat Kuwait in the final game of that group but eventually managed 1–0.

We then progressed into a three-team group with Germany and Spain hoping to qualify for the semi-finals. This was the first time and the last time this system was used to decide which teams go through to the semi-finals. I'm not surprised it was never used again because it became quite tactical. We had a goalless draw against Germany but then had to beat Spain by two goals to get through. We drew 0–0 with Spain and failed to qualify for the semi-finals. That game against Spain is well remembered as Kevin Keegan came on with ten minutes to go. Kevin had been suffering with a back problem and his playing was rusty. He missed a chance he probably would have normally scored with. Trevor Brooking was another player struggling with injury at the time. I'm still convinced if we had had Kevin Keegan and Trevor Brooking match-fit and at their best for that tournament we might easily have won the World Cup. We conceded only one goal in five games and didn't lose a single match. We just lacked that extra bit of flair which would have got us over the line. It was a strange feeling to have come home from a World Cup unbeaten.

My time at Forest was coming to an end. The successful team that won two European Cups was breaking up and new players were coming in. We weren't the same team as we had been, and I felt that the atmosphere had changed. So, when Southampton, under Lawrie McMenemy, made an offer which was accepted by Forest, I was pleased to join. Big Lawrie was a big name in football and TV circles. He always kept Southampton in the news. Ironically, when I joined Southampton Kevin Keegan, having fallen out with Lawrie, had just left to join Newcastle United. Striker Mick Channon had also left six months before to join Manchester City. After I'd played just a few games for the club, Alan Ball retired from football. Ball, Channon and Keegan had been a famous trio at Southampton, and they were no longer there. But we did have some talented young players like Mark Wright, the Wallace brothers, Steve Moran. And Southampton still boasted top players like Steve Williams, David Armstrong. Meanwhile, Matt Le Tissier and Alan Shearer were proving to be assets in our pretty decent youth team.

In my five years at Southampton, we reached two FA Cup semi-finals (against Everton and Liverpool respectively), one League cup semi-final (against Liverpool) and we finished runners-up in the First Division. Although we didn't actually *win* anything, I look on it as a very successful spell in my career.

During my time on the south coast, Lawrie McMenemy left for Sunderland. Lawrie did ask me to go with him, but I was happy with the Saints. It was a good decision on my part as unfortunately things didn't work out for him in the north-east. Chris Nicol, who was the centre half when I joined, took over as manager and did a very good job, he was a well-respected and honest professional.

It was whilst I was at the Dell that I played in my second World Cup in '86 in Mexico.

After the World Cup in Spain, Ron Greenwood had retired and Bobby Robson had taken over, keeping Don Howe as his assistant and bringing in Mike Kelly as a coach. Bobby soon confirmed my position as number one goalkeeper and my old friend and rival Ray Clemence decided to retire from international football. I played in the first ten matches under Bobby Robson and even wore the captain's armband in seven of those in the absence of Bryan Robson and Ray Wilkins. During that spell, a 2–0 win over Scotland in the Home International Championships saw me reach my 50th cap – a great landmark.

WORLD CUP '86 – THE HAND OF GOD

Before the World Cup in '86, the entire England squad went to Colorado Springs for a month to train and prepare for the altitude and heat we would be playing in when we arrived in Mexico. Bobby Robson warned us that we would have to over-train every day to get used to the conditions. It was gruelling. Sometimes we would come in, take our kit off and find puddles of sweat on the floor. We trained for two hours at a time. It was hard work, but worth it. We were very fit by the time we got to Mexico. Everything that could have been done, had been done to prepare for that World Cup. We arrived in Mexico a week or so before the first game and we were billeted, as in Spain, with our own armed guards. We were staying in bandit country.

We played out first game against Portugal in a stadium which I can only say was like a third division ground in England. Only three sides had space for spectators. The dressing rooms were reached via steps leading from the pitch behind one of the goals. The pitch was awful – very lumpy – and because of that they had let the grass grow too long to try to compensate. There were 5,000 spectators for that first game and absolutely no atmosphere at all. We really struggled to get going in that game. To make matters worse, Bryan Robson had to come off after injuring his shoulder and Ray Wilkins got send off for allegedly throwing the ball at the referee. We lost the game 1–0 which wasn't the start that we wanted. Our second match was not much better. We struggled to get a no score draw with Morocco. The media back home were starting to bay for blood.

Fortunately, our third game, which we *had* to win, against Poland turned things around. This game was played in a much bigger stadium which I was far more used to playing in. It had a descent surface and a there was a good crowd. We started a bit nervously. One of the Polish players got clean through our defence, but I managed to get down to block the shot and Terry Butcher knocked the ball back to me. That game became celebrated for Gary Lineker's hat-trick, which he has always said made his career. It was such a relief to get that result and move into the last sixteen. Our next game was played in the Aztec stadium against Paraguay, and we comfortably secured a 3–0 win. We were settling into the tournament. The next match was the crunch game against Argentina and their star player, Diego Maradona. It was the first game that Argentina and England had played against each other since the Falklands War of 1982 so it's no surprise that the build-up was huge and tense. Before the game, both camps did their best to play down the politically charged tensions before the big tie. Diego Maradona told the media that the game had nothing to do with the conflict over the Falklands and Bobby Robson said the same in his press conference prior to the match. They both emphasised that it was about the football and nothing to do with politics. The politics didn't enter my head but, however much Maradona and others tried to play it down, there was a definite edge to the game. We could all feel it. It probably meant more to Argentina. Their pride was at stake. They also had Diego Maradona who could win any game, all on his own and at any time.

In the absence of Bryan Robson and Ray Wilkins, I was made captain. I knew this England team was good enough to win the World Cup and the big hurdle was Argentina and Maradona in this quarter final. Argentina had Diego but we had Gary Lineker in red hot form and always likely to score. My thoughts were firmly fixed on winning that game so I could lead England into a World Cup Final.

It was a great atmosphere in the Aztec. We didn't make any strategic decisions on man-to-man marking of Maradona. Whoever was closest to him would close him down quickly. This worked well in the first half and we kept him quiet. It was an even game that saw no goals by half-time.

Seven minutes into the second half came the moment I will never forget. Maradona played a one-two on the edge of our box and went for a return pass. He would have been four or five yards offside, if one of his teammates had made the pass to him. But unfortunately, England's Steve Hodge was caught off balance whilst trying to clear the ball. Hodge knocked the ball backwards towards our goal. I had to make a decision. Should I stay on my line and let Maradona have an open goal from ten or twelve yards or try to get there before him. My split-second decision to leave my line was made on instinct. Maradona had momentum and I had to go from a standing start, but I reckoned I could get there just before him. I was at full stretch and had to make a long lunge at the ball just to try and knock it away with an outstretched fist. A striker's first instinct is to head the ball, and make it count. Maradona punched it. He clearly knew he wasn't going to achieve the header and opted to punch it and hope he could get away with it. I suspect it never crossed his mind that it wouldn't be spotted by the officials.

How referee, Ali Bin Nasser from Tunisia, and his assistant didn't see it, I will never know. Where was VAR when you needed it? The Argentine goal was allowed. I felt sick to my stomach when I saw the referee and officials racing to the centre circle ready to restart when it was obvious to the watching world that the goal had been scored with a handball. Some of the England players including Terry Fenwick and Glenn Hoddle pleaded with the referee, but he wasn't going to change his mind. Later the referee and his assistant blamed the other for missing the foul. Bin Nasser didn't officiate in another international match, and it would be hardly surprising if he did after the magnitude of that mistake.

Maradona's second goal of the match is rated one of the World Cup's best ever and it was, in my opinion, a wonderful goal. It demonstrated all the dribbling skills that we knew he possessed. His talent was incredible especially when you knew exactly how bumpy the pitch was. Not only did it show his great skill with the ball but his quickness of thought. However, that goal should never have been allowed as there was a blatant foul on Glenn Hoddle after a pass from Peter Beardsley ten yards inside our half before Maradona gained possession. The ref, who was right on top of the action, put the whistle to his mouth but, instead of blowing up as he should have done, he waved play on. Again, we protested, but it seemed we were destined not to get what we deserved in that match. The loose ball broke to Maradona and the rest is history. I also believe that, as a team, we were thrown by the unfairness of that first disputed goal, so we were not mentally tuned-in for the rest of that match.

We played on with John Barnes coming up from the bench and, along with Glenn Hoddle, setting up Gary Lineker to score. In the last few minutes Barnsie set up Gary Lineker again with another great cross. Gary looked as though he was certain to equalise with a close-range header, but he was pushed in the back by an opposition player. It should have been a penalty but again the referee missed it. Yet another decision that went against us. Gary insists to this day he was pushed and even now we all feel robbed. There's no doubt in my mind that we were cheated out of a chance to win that World Cup.

Bobby Robson was as shell-shocked as the rest of us when he came into the dressing room. "He did handle it, didn't he?" the England manager said to himself as much as to us. We told him that yes, we had all seen Maradona score with a handball. Robson turned round and left. I've no idea if he stormed off see the ref, but I wouldn't have blamed him if he had! The atmosphere in that England dressing room was the worst I have ever experienced in my entire career – and it's been quite a long career! It was most definitely the angriest dressing room I've ever been in. We were all in a state of sheer disbelief mixed with fury. Some of the squad were angry with the ref, some were angry with Maradona. I just sat there, stunned. I couldn't quite believe the way the game had gone. It wasn't very pleasant, but we couldn't do anything to change the result. We'd tried protesting on the pitch but there was no point in doing that now. Where would it have got us? Nowhere. Probably into a lot of bother. There wasn't a thing we could do apart from accept the result.

Terry Butcher was picked out to have a random drug test a few hours after that match. He told me that Maradona burst into the room still celebrating. Butch didn't speak Spanish, so he used hand gestures and signals to ask him whether he had scored with his head or his hand. Diego pointed at his head. Did he really believe that was the truth?

Steve Hodge had asked for and been given the shirt Diego Maradona wore in that game. I didn't see him go into the dressing room to ask it. No one would have been happy with him if we had. In fact, we would have been fuming and would probably have told him to take it back. Apparently, back at the hotel Hodgie pulled the shirt out of his kit bag and showed it to his roommate, Peter Reid. When we found out, Hodgie told us that he hadn't seen the handball incident, so didn't realise anything was wrong!

Years later, I saw Ali Bin Nasser hugging Maradona when he was on a trip to Tunisia. I was infuriated. I think that summed the whole thing up.

If I were the referee who had made such a massive mistake I would have kept as far away from Maradona as possible.

Just recently, I was watching a re-run of that infamous quarter-final game in Mexico as part of the 30th anniversary of Italia '90. Alongside it they were also showing some significant retrospective footage including commentary from football veterans like Jack Charlton. They brought on Terry Venables, one of ITV's star pundits at the time. What he said about that fateful goal in Mexico surprised me. Terry stated that I should have "cleaned him (Maradona) out" that is that I should have stopped him anyway I could – legitimate or not – just clattered into him and hoped for the best. I couldn't believe it. Terry Venables is a coach and a manager who I had much admired throughout my career. To hear this suggestion from a real "football man" was shocking to me. If you study the incident closely it's clear that, given a few extra seconds, I would have jumped higher than Maradona and cleared the ball comfortably. Not long after the game, a friend said to me, "Pete, if you chop off Maradona's left arm, you were definitely getting to the ball first," which I thought sums up the incident perfectly. So, I was surprised to hear Terry Venables suggest that I should have fouled him. I'm not sure giving away a penalty and being sent off would have been a clever option. What also surprised me was that Venables didn't lay any blame on Maradona. He seemed to ignore the fact that Maradona had got away with a handball. His actions had cheated England out of the World Cup but all I could see was Venables pointing an accusing finger in my direction! Terry's comments really rubbed salt further into the wounds left by that match.

A few years ago, I was invited out to the Far East to do some TV work and was told Maradona was managing a team out there. It was clear that they wanted to entice me to meet him. I made it clear to the organisers that I was happy to go out there, but that I would not be meeting Maradona and certainly not shaking his hand unless he was ready to offer up an apology. I was taken to the match where Diego's team was playing in Abu Dhabi. It was a 60,000-seater, state-of-the-art stadium. But with a crowd of only about 2,000 people in it. Half of those were paid to make an atmosphere – a rent-a-crowd all congregated into a tiny section, continuously chanting away. The atmosphere was pretty poor for such a large stadium They placed me in a seat that couldn't have been closer to the dugout where Maradona was sat. We were no more than 50 yards away, and I knew the intent was to get a picture of the two of us as close together as possible. As hard as they tried, they failed to get that picture. I was determined not to be seen near him. Peter Reid was also invited on that trip and he was pictured in the press shaking Diego's hand. That really did astonish me as Terry Butcher, Peter and myself were the most vociferous in condemning Diego.

I was also invited to go out to Argentina to meet Maradona, to appear on his chat show, with an offer of a very high fee to do it. But I didn't trust him to treat me properly, and so turned it down flat. In 2007, Gary Lineker had organised to interview Maradona for a film he was making twenty years after the match in Mexico. I was told that Gary had been messed around by Maradona who didn't turn up at the agreed time. When Gary first met Diego, he couldn't resist asking him which hand he used during a jokey exchange. In the clip, Lineker is seen shaking hands with Maradona before asking him: "Which hand was it? This one?" Maradona responded with a laugh lifted his left arm up, replying, "No, it was this one!"

During that interview, Gary asked Maradona more directly about the goal. Maradona said: "It was my hand. With this I don't mean any disrespect to English fans, but this is something that happened. We used to do this. I had scored goals before in Argentina with my hand. It was a goal that… I couldn't reach it and Shilton was already there, so I couldn't head it. So, I did like that (raising his left hand toward the side of his head) and I move my head back. And I started running because Shilton didn't realise. The one who told him, he was the sweeper, he was the one who sees my hand … When I see the linesman running I go out shouting, 'Goal'. I look behind me to see whether the referee took the bait. And he had! So, that was it. Come on, come on it was a goal! No, I don't think it's cheating. It's cunning. It's cheekiness. It can be handling the ball or… No, no, it's not cheating. I don't think it's cheating. I believe it's a craftiness. Maybe we have a lot more of it in south America than in Europe, but… it's not cheating. Because God gives us a hand. Because He gave us a hand. Because it is very difficult for it not to be seen by two people, the referee and the linesman, so that's why I said it was the hand of God incident."

This was the first time I had heard Maradona admitting so much about this incident and it was enlightening for me. I felt vindicated that what I had been saying about for 35 years was true. He confessed that he handled it because he was not going to make it to the ball before me. He had knowingly cheated to score that goal. I don't think cheating is down to interpretation or that the rules somehow don't matter in South American football. For me, and for football in England, fair play is important and respected. Cheating is not clever. Cheating is cheating no matter how you dress it up or try to explain it. It is taking advantage or manipulating the rules or trying to get round the rules. Maybe it goes on all the time in South America and not much is made of it. Maybe a player's entire career can be built around it. But there couldn't be a more high-profile incident than this. Where the eyes of the world were upon you and you chose to cheat in order to win.

Diego still stopped short of an apology, in fact he actually said he had nothing to apologise for. A player of Diego's stature could have apologised, that's the least he could have done.

Just before the last World Cup, I was approached by an agent who wanted to set up a promotional advertisement and a tour for Maradona and myself. We were both offered a lot of money to do it – a lot of people desperately wanted to see us shake hands and put a line under the Hand of God goal, once and for all. I made it clear to the negotiators that I would not participate unless Maradona agreed to apologise to me and to the country. I received the message back that he had flatly refused stating he would "never apologise" to me or my country. I knew then and there that a reconciliation would never take place in our lifetimes – it was never going to happen. He was the best player I ever played against on the pitch, but I had no respect for him off it.

While writing this book, a journalist contacted me to tell me that rumours were circulating in Argentina that Diego Maradona was dead. Fifteen minutes later, it was officially confirmed that Diego Maradona had died at the age of 60. I was immediately inundated with media requests from around the world inviting me to discuss one of the most infamous World Cup incidents in the history of the game. Obviously I was deeply shocked to hear of Diego's death, but sadly, I was not surprised. I knew that, a few weeks earlier, he had undergone very serious brain surgery, and clearly his health was not great. Like everyone, I knew he had an erratic lifestyle and had been concerned that this lifestyle would eventually catch up with him. I had feared the worst for my old adversary. Even so, it was still quite a shock when I received the call. I was sad, because the guy was only 60. I felt for his family. The whole of the football world was in shock, and it was devastating for the whole of Argentina. Despite our history, I tweeted my condolences to his family. The media was only interested in hearing about our differences, but I genuinely felt sorry for the loss of this great footballer.

ITALIA '90

I don't know if it was just the right time or that I had the five-year itch, but Arthur Cox from Derby County made a bid for me and it was an offer too good to refuse. I found myself back in the East Midlands. Robert Maxwell had just taken over as chairman at Derby. Arthur Cox and Stuart Webb had come down to my house in Southampton to talk to me about me coming to the club and what sort of terms I would want. Afterwards, I had been invited to Robert Maxwell's penthouse office at the *Mirror* to conclude the deal. I got on well with Robert Maxwell. It seemed to me that he wasn't worried about the terms but more about making sure he got it in the sports headlines of the *Mirror* the next day.

He had big ambitions for the club, which had just gained promotion to the First Division. While the Baseball Ground wasn't a big stadium, at least the pitch had improved from the days under Dave Mackay. Maxwell saw my move as a big signing for Derby County and promised me there would be more signings. Quite soon after I joined, he signed Mark Wright, my teammate from Southampton. I had recommended Mark. I played behind him when he was an inexperienced youngster at Southampton, and he had developed into a terrific player. Also, I liked him a lot. Quite a few big clubs were interested in him at the time, but I persuaded him to join me at Derby. He said afterwards that the fact I would be playing behind him was one of the big motivations to join the team. I went on to play behind him for England and we were always a good team together. He was a tall lad, great in the air, but besides being a

SAVED

good defender, he was also a good all-round footballer. Maxwell, at that time, true to his word also signed Dean Saunders.

It all went very well to start with at Derby and we finished fifth in the league in our first season. I really enjoyed playing under Arthur Cox, he was very "old school" in terms of the way he approached football. He was down to earth. He had previously been at Newcastle United and had taken Kevin Keegan to St. James's. I particularly liked his no-nonsense way of talking. He had a sense of humour and, at times, he needed it! I really enjoyed Arthur's training style – it was not complicated but it was effective. I especially enjoyed his Thursday morning squad shooting and finishing sessions, which were great for me as a goalkeeper. It was a valuable extra to me undertaking the specialised training with the other keepers on the squad. I did very little on Fridays after the heavy Thursday sessions. Whereas the other players had a quiet 8-a-side game, I would do the warm-up, go back to the ground and have a nice soak in the bath. It meant I could get my energy back for the next day – match day.

During those days, I was often in discussion with another great, no-nonsense football man, Jimmy Sirrel. Jimmy was a friend of Arthur's and did some scouting and a bit of training for the club on Fridays. Jimmy loved a chat and always used to try to come into the bathroom when I had just got into the bath. Anybody who knew Sirrel will remember that he had a very broad Scottish accent. I honestly hardly understood what he was saying and would spend nearly an hour nodding and agreeing with him from the bathtub without having a clue what he was talking about.

Things started to go downhill at Derby as suddenly the investment money dried up. I recall Arthur Cox telling me that he wanted to pay £600,000 for a player – not expensive for a player in those days – but Robert Maxwell refused to put up the cash. It was not quite the same at the club. We hardly saw Maxwell attending games and he left his two sons to oversee the club. It was puzzling at the time but, when Maxwell's money problems came to light, it all became clear.

One game sticks out in my memory from my days playing for Derby. It was when we played away against Newcastle – Arthur Cox's old club. It was one of Paul Gascoigne's first matches for Newcastle, and Gazza absolutely ran the show that day, showing all the strength and great ability that made him such a brilliant player. We were overrun at times, but I still had one of the best games of my career, stopping at least three one-on-ones and making a number of other saves. It ended as a no-score draw but, to this day, Newcastle fans remind me of that performance. It must have been good because Arthur Cox, not known for his exuberance or emotions, asked me if he could keep my shirt after the game. I felt it was an honour that Arthur asked me, but the problem was that we only had one set of kit for the entire season in those days. So the club had to find a new shirt for me for the next game. How times have changed. Players get a new set of kit for every game – sometimes at half-time!

Another highlight of that time was playing for England in the Italia '90 World Cup. The build-up to Italia '90 was totally different to '86, because this time we didn't have to prepare for the extreme heat or the altitude. We gathered as a squad two weeks before the tournament started on the island of Sardinia. We stayed at a lovely hotel on a beach. Bobby Robson allowed players' wives to come over to spend a bit of time, just a few days, as they had had a long season. Bobby Robson was getting a lot of criticism back home in the papers, not only because of our match results in the build-up, but also about his past personal life. This was something that we players thought was disgraceful, and it made us even more determined to do well in the tournament.

Sardinia was a beautiful island and Bobby Robson took the squad to a fabulous restaurant one evening. We all enjoyed a great Italian meal and a few drinks. It broke the monotony and was a break away from the rigours of the preparation and hard training we were doing. The island was not the ideal place to start a World Cup as it was a fairly relaxing holiday island, and we players didn't quite feel the same as we might have done on the mainland in terms of the atmosphere and build up to the tournament.

Finally, the day of the first game was upon us and we were off and running against Jack Charlton's Republic of Ireland. That match brought back memories, not pleasant ones, of playing against the Republic of Ireland. We had lost 1–0 to them in the European Champions in Germany in 1988, with a Ray Houghton header. England didn't do very well in that tournament. I was captain when we played Holland in my

100th game for my country. Unfortunately, the game ended in a 3–1 defeat for us, which tempered my celebration.

That day in 1990 it had been raining before the match and it was still very windy – conditions you wouldn't have expected in Italy in June. As I lined up on that blustery day, I had to remind myself that I was actually at the World Cup. Looking at the Irish team and seeing the lads I played against week in and week out in such British-feeling weather conditions – I could have kidded myself that I was still at home. We knew that Ireland would play a direct game and use a lot of a long balls – totally different to any of the other teams in the competition. The game proved to be a difficult one, but I think the 1–1 draw was probably a fair result for both teams.

Our second match against Holland was quite different. It was end to end a proper football match as you would expect, and our performance was a lot better than against the ROI. Holland probably edged the possession, but we were unlucky not to end up winning the game. Stuart Pearce scored from a free kick only to have it disallowed. Next, we needed to beat Egypt to qualify. Despite dominating the game, we struggled to score until Mark Wright went up for a Gazza free kick in the final minutes and headed the ball home. What a relief. People may have forgotten that, just before we scored, Egypt had a great chance with an open goal from twelve yards out. The striker hit it sharply but not as well as he should have done. He *should* have scored, but it gave me the chance to get down sharply and make a save. We ended up winning 1–0 which saw us through to the last sixteen, but I often look back and think everything could have been so different – we could have been going home, if that strike had gone in.

We arrived in Bologna for the tie with Belgium. We were never able to see much of the towns we played in as we would be preparing for the match. But I remember walking out to inspect the ground before this tie and being amazed. It was unlike any other football stadium I had previously played in. It was so artistic and impressive – typical Italian architecture.

The players loved Bobby and we all respected him, but Bobby Robson liked a team meeting, and they did go on a bit. The lads used to call him "Mogadon" after the sleeping pill because you wouldn't need one after one of his team meetings. Before the Belgium game he held one of his all-time record length team meetings before we left for the ground. Thinking that was all over and done with, we then left for the match. At the stadium, players have their individual routines: some like to leave it until the last minute before they change into their kit and some like to change to give themselves plenty of time to go out and warm-up. Those of us who opted to get changed first went out for a warm-up. When we returned to the dressing room some of the players were just starting to get changed. Bobby came in, sat us all down and started the team meeting all over again – making virtually all the same points one more time. I was thinking "Christ, this is going to turn into another of Bobby's massive team meetings." It had already going on far longer than any of us would have liked and our "curtains" came down. Gazza never listened to Bobby's team talks at the best of times, and I could see him drifting off into a little world of his own. The rest of the players were also looking around at each other, perplexed. Then they started looking to me as the senior player in that dressing room. They wanted Bobby to wrap it up – they were beginning to lose concentration on what he was saying anyway. Some had not finished getting changed and wanted to get ready for the match. "Excuse me, boss…" I started to say. Then, Bobby looked at his watch and said: "OK, lads, I'll finish off now then. I think I lost all track of time."

The Belgium game was end to end and both myself and the Belgian keeper had quite a bit to do. I was pleased with my performance. Although Belgium hit the bar and the post I always made people smile when I say I never thought the shots were going to go in. Sometimes, as a goalkeeper, you *sense* things and during that match I knew the balls weren't on target. As we neared the end, both teams seemed resigned to a penalty shoot-out. But the final result has become famous because, in the last minute of extra time, Gazza took a free kick and lined up one of the greatest finishes of World Cup history. Gazza bent a great kick into the area where David Platt somehow acrobatically hooked the ball from behind him into the far corner of the Belgium net. Their keeper was given no chance. It was one of those great feelings, as a footballer, that you always remember. Belgium never had a chance to come back at us and we were through to the quarter-finals.

153

Having spent Italia '90 playing on a team with Gazza, I can tell you that all the hype and stories about him are true. I have seen the mischievous side of his character. Not only was he a terrific player, but he also had a cheeky, comical side. He was always on the go – you had no idea what he was going to do next, but you *did* know it would be something completely daft and unexpected. Everyone has stories about Gazza, but my favourite was watching his antics during our World Cup qualifier in Albania. At that time, Albania was quite a mysterious country for the rest of the world as they hardly ever opened its borders to anyone. So, it was a big occasion for the country to host the England team. The day before the game we went to the stadium to have a training session behind closed doors. Bobby Robson wanted us to practise our set plays, free kicks and corners in private. A number of the locals wanted to see the England team train. We had been training for about five or ten minutes when, suddenly, around 3,000 locals poured into the stadium to watch us. Bobby was not amused. He had been assured that security wouldn't allow anybody in, and he wanted to ensure our tactics were kept secret from the opposition. "Right," he hollered, "we are not doing set plays."

Training in the stadium should have been pretty routine, but things rarely were routine – not with Gazza around. At the end of training, I had done as much as I wanted to in preparation for the game. A group, including Gary Lineker, Chris Waddle and Gazza wanted to do some shooting practise. Chris Woods went in goal. The local fans were ecstatic to see Gazza, and he played up to the watching crowd. As he ran up to take his shot he waved his arms to get the crowd shouting, and they were only too happy to give him encouragement. The moment he made the shot he would motion his finger across his lips for the fans to be silent. You could hear a pin drop. They did exactly as Gazza motioned them to do. He was leading them like a conductor leads an orchestra. It was silly, but typical Gazza. He made shots at goal again and again, and the fans reacted to it exactly the same. They loved every minute of it. All of the players, myself included, were in fits of laughter watching this unfold. Only Gazza could have done something like that.

Next up in the competition for us was the surprise team in the tournament, Cameroon, who we were set to face in the great football city of Naples. It was totally different feel to Bologna, a bigger stadium and great atmosphere. We were told before the game by one of Bobby Robson's scouts that the Cameroons were a big, physical team but that we should beat them comfortably. How wrong that prediction turned out to be. Although we were clear favourites for the game, we soon realised that they were a good team. Early on, I had to face a one-on-one situation with a Cameroon player and managed to win that battle by blocking the shot. It was a wake-up call for us; this team could play. From then on, there was no holding back by both teams. It was end to end and must have been a great match to watch. I suppose the Cameroons, despite being strong and skilful, were a bit naive when it came to tactics but that didn't stop them causing a lot of problems for us in the game. We went 1–0 up with a goal from David Platt assisted by a great run and cross from Stuart Pearce down our left side. The game flowed end to end and I was having more action than in any game in the tournament up to now. Unfortunately, Gazza gave away a penalty. The shot was struck fiercely and high to my left and although I got a slight finger to it, the pace was too much. The Cameroons opened up our defence again and I was left one-on-one, twelve yards out. This time the player, Eugene Ekeke, kept his cool and put a great finish in the top corner. Thankfully, the Cameroons showed their naivety when defending by giving away two penalties in quick succession. Gary Lineker converted the first. And the second he shot straight down the middle, but the goalkeeper had moved early. We won 3–2 and felt our luck had changed. Things were going our way.

Next stop was Turin to face the Germans in a semi-final. There is always a massive build up to semi-finals, but an England vs. Germany match meant there was even more pressure.

Initially, I felt I was having a good game and made some great saves. Then Germany were awarded a free kick. I was on my line ready for whichever direction the ball might come at the goal – over the wall or straight at me. Andreas Brehme knocked it square, so I came out a few yards to narrow the angle. But the ball took a wicked deflection off of Paul Parker as he tried to block the shot, and it deflected more or less over my head into the net. I was caught square on facing the shot, which would have been the right position. But with the ball deflected over my head I needed to be sideways on, so I could use my feet quickly and jump into it. It was one of those things that goalkeepers can't legislate for – a complete fluke. I was gutted that Germany had taken the lead. As the game continued end to end, I knew that I didn't want us to lose by such a fluke, so I was pretty pleased when Gary Lineker equalised in the 59th minute. Paul Parker played a long pass to Gary and the Germans muddled their defence. Gary Lineker did what Gary Lineker was great at and stuck the ball into the bottom corner of the net. You could feel the relief go right through our entire team. Later, somebody told me that just before the goal, Bobby Robson had been warming up Steve Bull to come on in place of Gary. They quickly told him to sit down!

At one goal each, we went into extra time and, after five minutes, I made one of my best World Cup saves – a bullet of a header from Jürgen Klinsmann from only eight yards out. It was during extra time that we saw one of the most infamous moments for England football. Gazza, who carried a booking into the game having been yellow carded earlier in the tournament, lunged into a reckless tackle on Thomas Berthold. The lads later said that Berthold started whining and rolling around on the floor after the tackle. Gazza leaned over him and tried to put his hand across his mouth to stop him screaming as he knew the noise he was making would get him booked but it was to no avail. Gazza was given a yellow card. It meant he would miss the final if we got there. Suddenly the camera zoomed in on Gazza full of tears and Gary Lineker gesturing to the bench to keep an eye on his teammate. That was an unforgettable piece of TV which we have seen replayed time and time again. It must have been devastating at that moment for Gazza to realise his fate.

Extra time came to an end. The score was still 1–1. And so, the game went to penalties. Over the years I had faced a lot of penalties. One memorable one was when I played for Leicester in the fifth round of the FA Cup at Liverpool in 1969. I saved a penalty in front of the Kop, against Tommy Smith. We went on to get to the Cup Final that year. But this was my first penalty shoot-out. The Germans, on the other hand, had a great reputation in penalty shoot-outs.

My strategy had always been to avoid committing myself too early and diving the wrong way. This is a mistake a lot of keepers make. Because of the pressure on the penalty takers, they are more likely to hit straight at the goalie. So, I waited as long as I could before committing myself, playing the percentages.

Gary Lineker scored with the first penalty for England. The first penalty-taker for Germany was Andreas Brehme. I'd saved one against him in a previous game with Germany when he shot to my left. I figured he would remember that and would change sides and shoot to my right. Although I guessed correctly he hit it with pace just inside the post. Peter Beardsley made it 2–1 to England. Lothar Matthäus equalised for Germany – again shot to my right and with immense pace. David Platt gave us 3–2 for England with Karlheinz Riedle equalising again for the opposition. Uncharacteristically Stuart Pearce more or less hit his penalty straight at their goalkeeper, Bodo Illgner. Olaf Thon scored with Germany's fourth penalty. The pressure was on and some of the lads didn't want to take the penalties, but Chrissie Waddle stepped up. I remember saying to myself "Please score." Chris had played really great in the game but unfortunately his penalty went over the bar and we were out. In terms of anticipating the direction and angle of the German players' shots, I guessed right in all of the four penalties I faced. But they all went into the corner just inside the post – like rockets – giving me no chance to make a save. Every one was struck with power and precision.

We had been so close. It was the worst feeling going out on penalties when we were the better team. It had been my ambition to win the World Cup and that feeling of going out so close to the final was something hard, if not impossible, to describe. Of course, saying that, I and the whole squad were proud of our performance in Italia '90. It had rejuvenated football in our country and also it was the best any team had achieved since the World Cup win on our own soil in '66.

We still had the third and fourth place play-offs to play. Having just lost in the semi-final most teams don't want to play these matches – they just want to go home.

Our first play-off match against Italy in Bari would be my last England game as I had made the decision to retire, so I was team captain. It was a very windy day but a great atmosphere for that game because Italy were the home nation. I was pleased with my performance that day as I had quite a lot to do. But I was blamed for the first Italian goal. I was rolling the ball out, ready to distribute it to the side of my goal, when Roberto Baggio sneaked behind me and took the ball away. The ball went outside the box for a minute but eventually came back in. We had two or three opportunities to clear it, but it ended up in the back of our net. Losing possession of the ball was clumsy, but I don't look at it as a goalkeeping technique error. As it was my last game, I got the blame. Italy were then awarded a dubious penalty. In our eyes that shouldn't have happened. We thought the referee was what we would call a "homer" meaning he was influenced in favour of the home nation. Salvatore Schillaci scored, sending me the wrong way. Our luck – certainly my luck – had deserted us with those two dubious goals.

I had already decided, before the tournament began, that I was going to retire no matter what. I knew Bobby Robson was going to finish as manager and I was nearly 41 at the time and still playing for Derby County. After we beat Belgium, I told him that I had decided to retire when he stepped down as manager at end of the tournament. I'd heard indirectly that Graham Taylor who was taking over from Bobby Robson after the tournament, wanted me to still carry on. I felt I could have done that as I thought I'd had a good tournament, but my decision was made.

After twenty years in the game, playing for England in three World Cups and having the joint best record for goals conceded (ten in seventeen matches, shared with Fabien Barthez – if it weren't for the Hand of God, I'd have the record outright) I felt I wanted to go out on a high. I read that when Alan Shearer decided to retire, he felt the same. He felt that he may have been able to carry on longer but like myself, he decided that you get to a point when age starts to get used against you in football. When you leave yourself open to criticism – like myself and Alan did – any mistakes, any missed chances are because you are "too old". It's better to go out at the top on your own terms rather wait for somebody to push you.

After that last match against Italy, everyone just wanted to get home. And we were all blown away really by the reception we got after we landed at Luton airport. There were hundreds – maybe thousands – of people there to welcome us. That's when it really hit home for me just how well we had done. We didn't win the Cup but we went further than any other England team had done away from home and I'm very proud of that. When I arrived back in my village in Leicestershire there were 40 or 50 people waiting to clap me as I got out of my car. They had put flags up and all sorts. I couldn't believe it. They were showing me how well they thought the team had done.

Italia '90 brought the curtain down on my England career. I went out with 125 caps, a record at the time, and one that has yet to be beaten. Bobby Robson also came to the end of his tenure as England manager and Graham Taylor took over. Shortly afterwards, I got a call from Graham asking me to come along to coach the England goalkeepers. In July I was saying goodbye to England, and by September I was back coaching Chris Woods, David Seaman and my old England World Cup squad teammate, David Beasant. It was a bit surreal to say the least. I was still playing for Derby but being back around the England team didn't feel right. I still felt as though I was England's number one keeper. After seven months coaching, I decided that I had returned too quickly to the England squad. And I wasn't sure if I really wanted to go down the goalkeeping coaching route full time. I had got my eyes on a management role. I wanted a fresh challenge and, at the time, I think it was the right decision. Later, with hindsight and after my management career finished prematurely, I felt all my years of goalkeeping expertise, developing techniques and training exercises, *could* have been used in a valuable way. Maybe I should have carried on. I might still be England's goalkeeping coach now, who knows? Certainly, I will always look back with enormous fondness at my last World Cup in Italia '90, and that tournament will live with me for a lifetime.

Back at Derby, we had been relegated. The next season we were aiming for promotion. We had a good chance of bouncing back. Robert Maxwell had sold the club to local businessman Lionel Pickering who had invested in the club. But I was looking for a change. I felt that, even though we were doing quite well that season, I needed to start thinking about the future and that for me was management. Toward the end of that season the opportunity arose to become player-manager at Plymouth. And I took it.

I began what I thought would be a successful managerial career at Plymouth Argyle but it was not as easy an assignment as I'd anticipated. Geography, for a start: being so far south made it a challenge to bring in new players, especially from the north. Away games were always a challenge as the distances we needed to travel were often substantial.

When I took over as player-manager, the team were sitting second bottom of the league. We had three really decent players, Dwight Marshall was one of them. He had signed from a non-league side where he had scored most of goals. I decided to try to sign a striker to play with him and give him support on the pitch. The club backed me, and we signed Kevin Nugent from Leyton Orient, but unfortunately he quite quickly broke his big toe and was out for the season. We had to beat Blackburn Rovers, under Kenny Dalglish, in the last game of the season to stay up. Rovers were too much for us, they were too good a team – and we were relegated. Not the perfect start by any stretch of the imagination. I was convinced that had Nugent stayed fit he would have made a big difference.

The next season I started a rebuilding of the team, but funds were low. I managed to sign a young goalkeeper from Cheltenham Town, Alan Nichols, for £5,000. He developed so quickly that I could take a back seat and concentrate on managing. I sold two good players, Nicky Marker and Jock Morrison, to Kenny Dalglish at Blackburn for a combined fee of £1 million plus a couple of players in return including a centre half, Keith Hill, who has made quite a success in management in the north in the lower leagues and is a good character. With some of the money from the sale, I bought three or four players including Andy Comyn from Derby, a centre half who had previously played for Aston Villa. I also recruited Steve Castle from Leyton Orient; Paul Dalton, a left winger from Hartlepool and Steve McCall, a left back from Sheffield Wednesday who I played in midfield. I paid £25,000.

In my second full season, we topped the league for parts of the campaign, and ended up third place in the league, scoring more goals (85) than any team in all four divisions. We played attractive, attacking football in a style that people still speak to me about to this day. We regularly took gates of 18,000. Unfortunately, we just missed out on automatic promotion. We had beaten Hartlepool 8–1 in the final game of the season, but Port Vale had also won at Brighton meaning they got the final automatic slot. We finished twelve points ahead of Burnley, but they went on to win the play-off final.

Away from the football, I always had problems with my chairman Dan McCauley during my time at Plymouth. The first time I met the directors was at a venue on the outskirts of Ipswich where they interviewed me for the job. Plymouth were playing Ipswich the next day and I travelled down from the Midlands. I always remember that McCauley was the only director who was trying to be a bit clever but, at that time, I just ignored him. To me, he was a little man, who had little man's syndrome. He looked to try to upset people – it was just the way he was. I never really ever got on with him. I think, perhaps, the only time he seemed normal with me was when we were top of the league.

After our successful season, I had discussions with the directors about a new contract. The chairman wanted me to take a pay cut as we hadn't secured promotion. I wanted to keep working for the club and continue with the progression I had made, so I agreed. We had a disastrous run of injuries at the start of the season, losing Castle, who had scored 26 goals the previous season, with yellow jaundice, Paul Dalton, who had scored 15 goals with a broken leg, and Nuggent with a hamstring. Within six months we were struggling. In my eyes it was hardly surprising that, instead of winning games by the odd goal, we were losing them by the odd goal.

My relationship with the chairman had broken down and I left the club by mutual consent. I have to admit that some of the reasons were my own fault. But from a purely football point of view, and considering the bad run of injury problems, I considered my time there a success. The chairman had five managers in five years after I left. One of those managers was Neil Warnock who lasted just ten months. Warnock was a very experienced manager and even he couldn't work with McCauley. He was a very difficult man to work for.

Not all players who reach the top of their playing career, naturally become managers, but I had played for some of the top managers of their time and learned so much from them. I'd learned from people like Tony Waddington at Stoke, who bought me to the club for a record fee at that time. I rated Matt Giles very highly as my first manager – you couldn't wish for a better man to work under when you are just starting out in your football life. Of course, there was Brian Clough and Peter Taylor, it goes without saying that I learned so much from them. Then there was Lawrie

McMenemy at Southampton and Arthur Cox at Derby and of course, most of my England managers. It's often said that not many goalkeepers can make great managers. Well, that's a very old fashioned and blinkered view. There are numerous exceptions such as Dino Zoff and, more recently, Nuno Espírito Santo at Wolves. It's the same with being captain, many so-called experts think goalkeepers don't make good captains, but it's not a school of thought I would subscribe to. Goalkeepers can see the *whole* of the pitch during a game – all the action is taking place straight ahead of them. So I would think they often make better captains than say strikers.

Having been a bit isolated at Plymouth, I was determined to get back into the football world. I knew I had always kept myself fit and knew that, on a short-term basis, I could still perform goalkeeping at Premiership level. When I left Plymouth, I was on 996 league games, and I also thought it would be a great achievement to reach the 1,000 game mark and achieve that in the Premier League. If I did it, I would become the first player in the history of English football to play 1,000 League games so I set myself a new target.

My next club was Coventry City who had just gained promotion to Division One, with Big Ron Atkinson in charge. Their first-choice goalkeeper, Steve Ogrizovic was in the process of recovering from a broken leg, and their other keeper, John Phelan, was still relatively inexperienced. Big Ron wanted me as experienced back-up with a chance of playing if things didn't work out for the young keeper. Unfortunately, I didn't get the chance to play in the first team. Oggy returned to fitness and my time at Coventry was finished. However, it was whilst I was at Coventry that I recommended Big Ron take on my son, Sam, who was playing for Plymouth. He was only sixteen but had played in the first team a couple of times through our chronic injury crisis. Big Ron paid £20,000 for him and Sam went on to play in the first team a few times.

The next call I had was from Joe Kinnear at Wimbledon who had a goalkeeping crisis for an FA Cup tie at Anfield. Hans Segers had been taken ill and Joe signed me as cover. Although it wasn't a league game I was happy to help him out. I was looking forward to playing and doing battle with Liverpool at Anfield again. Hans Segers recovered at the last minute and played, so I didn't get the chance to play at Anfield again but watched from the bench.

Unknown to me at the time, Bruce Rioch, the Bolton manager, was in the crowd that day at Anfield and was watching as I warmed-up. Bolton were enjoying a very successful season, were due to play in the League Cup Final against Liverpool at Wembley and also in contention for promotion to the First Division. Bruce contacted me and said he would like me to join the club for the last three months of the season in case he had any problems with his two keepers, Keith Brannagan, a Republic of Ireland international, and Aidan Davison. I was still living down in the Plymouth area at the time, so I had to travel up and stay in the Bolton area all week. It was great to go back to Wembley for the Cup Final, but Liverpool won it.

I played two league games for Bolton when Keith Brannagan was injured. Aidan Davison played when we faced my old club, Stoke, and I was on the bench. Davison was sent off after only ten minutes after a foul on Paul Peschisolido which give a penalty away to the opposition. I went on and the first time I touched the ball was to pick it out of the net. Toddy Orlygsson sent me the wrong way and scored for Stoke. The next 80 minutes went much better for me, especially the second half where I made a number of good saves. At 46, I was the oldest to have played at the Victoria Ground, since Sir Stanley Matthews played when he was 50.

After my performance at Stoke, Bruce Rioch picked me to play for Bolton in the first leg of the play-off against Wolves, under Graham Taylor, at Molineux. It was a capacity crowd and although we lost 2–1 I had another very good game. So much so, that many Wolves and Bolton fans still comment on that performance when I encounter them. For the second leg, Keith Brannagan returned from injury and Bolton won 2–0 and got to the play-off final. That was game No. 996 and I was back at Wembley on the bench as Bolton made it to the Premier League by beating Reading 4–3 to gain promotion. And with that, I finished my time at the club. It was nice to have played a part and been involved with success at such a famous club.

The next phone call I had was from Harry Redknapp who wanted me to head to West Ham to coach his goalkeepers and be an experienced back-up keeper. Not long after I joined, Ludo Mikloško, his number one keeper, got injured and I was suddenly on standby. That Friday Harry twice told me I would be playing on Saturday in the first team, only to change his mind on Saturday morning. I played a couple of pre-season friendlies. I would have loved to play for them at Upton Park. I actually played couple of games to keep match fit in the reserves a couple of times and once I played with Rio Ferdinand at centre-half, Frank Lampard in midfield and Jermain Defoe up front. But, after one game for West Ham against my old club Forest, I decided it was probably the time to move on. I needed two more games. The opportunity came to go to Leyton Orient up the road. Les Sealy, who was their keeper, wanted to return to the Hammers to become their goalkeeping coach. So we swapped over.

My 1,000th match was on 22nd December 1996. Leyton Orient were playing at home to Brighton. The Football League wanted to make a presentation to me before the match and it was broadcast live on Sky TV, a rarity for an Orient fixture. The club did well financially out of the match. I did mention to the manager, Barry Hearn, that I didn't want anyone to go over the top with celebrations. He laid a red carpet from the tunnel, which stretched all the way to my area, and released 1,000 balloons to celebrate my 1,000th game. Not exactly downplaying it!

I kept a clean sheet and we won 2–0, although I didn't have that much to do in that match which was a touch disappointing because the previous week we had played Fulham at Craven Cottage and I had a great game which had ended in a 1–1 draw. I wish the performances had been reversed but maybe not the scores. I always had a soft spot for Leyton Orient as a club so, despite it being a lower level of football than I had played before, I was still happy to have broken the record there.

I ended up playing nine times, two of them in cup ties, for Orient. But it was now all over. I'd got to my 1,000th league game, and I knew it was time to finish as I wasn't really enjoying it any longer playing at that level. I knew it was the end of my playing career. No more targets. No more football. Football had been my life for 30 years, but it was now over. It's funny how life takes you in different directions and right now I am glad I am where I am, but it felt very bittersweet back then. I finished on a record-breaking note. But now I knew it was over.

I'm immensely proud of my achievements in football. I kept myself fit and 61 of my 125 caps were earned after my 35th birthday. In 1989 I broke Bobby Moore's record with my 109th appearance in a friendly

1–0 win over Denmark in the Danish centenary celebration match. I completed a career record 1,005 League appearances. I ended my playing career with a world record of competitive games played: 1,387 games for club and country in the history of football. I knew I had given 100 per cent whether in playing or training right through my 30-year record-breaking career.

RAY CLEMENCE

A SPECIAL TRIBUTE TO MY FRIEND AND ROOMMATE OF 10 YEARS

On 15th November 2020 I tweeted: "I'm absolutely devastated to be told of the sad news that Ray Clemence has just passed away. We were rivals but good friends. Ray was a brilliant goalkeeper with a terrific sense of humour. I will miss him a great deal as we've kept friends long after retiring. RIP, my friend."

When I heard of Ray's death I was devastated. Ray was an England teammate and a rival over the years but, more importantly, he was my friend. I knew he had been unwell and in hospital. We had exchanged texts and the last one I have from him was a "thumbs up" emoji. He did not want people to worry about him. That was typical of Ray. Back in the day, we were competitors, both aiming to be England's number one goalkeeper. But we always got on and we roomed together for ten years whilst on England duty. And the thing is, we never talked about football when we were together. Ray was a warm man with a great sense of humour and we would spend most of our time laughing. It was not frowned upon to socialise and even have a drink whilst on England duty back then, and we used to do that. He was great fun on a night out and those nights continued after we had both retired, with reunions, golf days and other get-togethers. It was always great to see him. He was one of those people you could trust and an all-round great guy. I'm just so sad he was taken from us so early in his life.

On the field, Ray was a very natural goalkeeper. He was tall, incredibly athletic and had great goalkeeping hands. Ray was totally reliable and unfussy. He was not showy or extravagant but, of his era, there were very few better. When I was at Nottingham Forest, he was playing for

Liverpool and there was great rivalry between the clubs. But for us, it never changed a thing. We were mates. When England manager Ron Greenwood made the decision to pick me over Ray for the 1982 World Cup squad, I know how I would have felt had I been in Ray's position. But he never let that disappointment or upset show. He just got on with it and I can't pay him any greater compliment than that really.

Ray got 61 caps for England. People sometimes say to me, "If Clem hadn't been around how many caps would you have got?" I always answer, "Listen, Ray was a fantastic goalkeeper and deserved the caps he got." I think Ray would admit that I was a more enthusiastic trainer than he was but, of course, he went on to be a very good and respected goalkeeping coach with England. Once before a big England game I was on the sidelines doing some work for Sky and Ray was on the pitch doing some work with Paul Robinson. I realised Ray was using one of the routines that I had devised. I shouted across to him, "Clem, you have nicked my drills, mate!" He just laughed and shouted back, "Sorry, Shilts!" That is how I will remember him. That big smile. I still can't believe he has gone at such a young age.

TRIBUTES

NEVILLE SOUTHALL

Peter Shilton was the first of a different generation of goalkeepers, someone who took goalkeeping on to a new level and pushed the boundaries further. He learned from Banksie (Gordon Banks) having been at the same club with him but then he took the art of goalkeeping further. He had incredible agility and fantastic reactions, but he was also a great presence, a good communicator and a good organiser – the complete package. In his day, he was unbeatable.

I've met Peter a few times and he's a really nice fellow. He has achieved a level of consistency that few others have done. I would say he learned from quite a few people during his years in the game, but none more so than Brian Clough during their time together at Nottingham Forest. Brian Clough allowed him to get on with things and be himself. In our day, there was no such thing as goalkeeping coaches so not only did he learn from others, but he also had to be largely self-taught. To play for as long as he did was remarkable, especially as he virtually coached himself. While it sounds easy enough to take in all that knowledge from so many people, it is the way you *use* that knowledge is the key. Shilts was someone who could take in all that information and not only apply it but learn and improve with the way he trained. His constant determination to improve helped him to become one of the best goalkeepers there has ever been. When I watch old footage of goalkeepers and see some of his saves, it makes me appreciate even more than I did at the time, just how good he was. There was really no one to touch him.

Modern day goalkeepers are light years behind him. You go back to Banks, Clemence, Shilton and you realise that goalkeepers are so vastly different these days. For example, keepers these days are taught to push the ball away from the goal, whereas we would catch it. We had some good goalkeepers and some outstanding ones, but today there are no *outstanding* goalkeepers. They have a vastly different mindset – maybe because they don't have the freedom that we enjoyed. There seems to be a focus on what you *can't* do, rather than what you *can* do. When you see goalkeepers knocking the ball away, you think, we would never have got away with that in our time. We would have been slaughtered. We moved to *hold* the ball, not push it away. It's a different way of thinking, and a different way of playing and that is why there are not too many great goalkeepers knocking about today. We set about wanting to be the best, by training harder than anyone, to prove that hard work pays off.

I've taken steps to tackle the issues of mental illness in football in my new book *Mind Games*. And it doesn't surprise me to hear that Shilts has opened up about his personal gambling addiction. It's commendable that he had the strength of character not to carry his personal issues onto the pitch, but for many that is impossible. Sometimes the pitch is the one place where footballers can escape personal problems but, once the game is over, those problems are still there. People on the outside simply don't realise how easy it is to fall into a trap. And those who have fallen into traps should not be ashamed of it, or ashamed to admit it and talk about it.

Gambling addiction in football is a controversial subject, because the public see footballers with their generous salaries and think it's easy for them to enjoy having a bet – they can afford to do so. They can walk onto a pitch and play without worrying about the sort of things that trouble people paid, on average, far less. We might have been top earners in our time – especially Peter – but in reality footballers then and today are not idols. We are normal people albeit ones the fans love to watch play football, and we suffer pressures as much as anyone – sometimes too much pressure. People in the game have not got to grips about how players can chill out, relax, away from the game, and too often they end up with an addiction, and in the case of gambling those £50 bets can mount up far too easily. The temptation is there, and it can easily get out of hand. The football industry hasn't got to grips with the pressures on players, the sudden shock of having more than enough money for many young players and the desire to escape that pressure during their downtime. The conditions are all too perfect for cultivating gambling addictions. And just because the cash flow is there it doesn't mean those addictions can't get out of hand and become destructive.

It's much harder for the modern player to escape the pressures of the game now. We didn't have mobile phones but there is no escaping social media now. This opens players up to direct, sometimes harsh criticism from fans. Trust has been lost. The pressure from the media can be overwhelming. I've always felt that the media put a great deal of focus on the England team and that's spread to social media.

It can only help, the game, the fans and society, when someone as respected as Peter Shilton comes out and tells it like it is – how it really is. To open up about his struggle with addiction and explain how he came through it. Of course, being a Labour voter, I don't like the fact that he's a Tory, but I can only admire Peter for doing that. I really like what he is doing there.

CHRIS WOODS

If you were to ask me about Peter Shilton, I would have to say that, for me, he was the best technical goalkeeper in the world. Technically, he had all the attributes you need for a goalkeeper. He worked hard on every aspect of goalkeeping. In terms of agility, he was so quick – the way he would get down to make saves and how his arms seemed a lot longer because he was able to reach shots it seemed impossible to. The way he trained was an eye-opener for me, and it was a privilege to be there and watch him train. He wanted his training to be perfect. He had a remarkable determination, on the training ground and he took that into matches. He'd work hard throughout the week and train the most intensely on a Thursday before a Saturday game. Friday was always the day he would set aside for his recuperation from the hard week of training in preparation for the match day. There were days in training, when we had shooting drills. During those, he was just unbelievable – you couldn't actually get a single shot past him. I learned so much when I trained with him during our England years. He was a goalkeeper I looked up to, one I always wanted to emulate if I could. I wanted to replicate the dedication, hard work and focus he put into his training every day. In a match there was nothing that could happen that would affect his playing.

Playing against a team with Peter on it was tough. He would make the sort of saves that left you in awe. "Here we go, we are in for one of those afternoons" you would think. You would feel a strange certainty that your side would have do something really outstanding to beat him. And, as opposition goalkeeper, if you made a save, you couldn't help wondering what he thought of it!

For me, one of Peter's great attributes was that he was always switched on and always one step ahead. Most keepers would be wondering what would be the best course of action as a cross comes into the box, but Shilts would already be thinking "What happens next?" He was alert to everything.

The fact that he won 125 caps for his country, a record that has not been broken in the 30 years since he set it, speaks volumes for his ability. It is just an unbelievable record. During Italia '90 play-offs, Bobby Robson told me I'd play on the England squad but then Shilts announced he was going to retire, and he played in that final match against Italy, earning his 125th cap. In no way would I hold that against him, he deserved that last game.

In recent years, we met up not so long ago at St. George's Park on a goalkeepers' course. Rather than listen to a presentation on gloves, I opted out to spend 45 minutes chatting with Shilts. That meant far more to me than listening to a chat about gloves! We spoke about all sorts of things like how we both saw goalkeepers of the current generation of footballers. There was a time when we had the best goalkeepers in the world and Shilts was the perfect example. But that isn't the case now. We chatted about the reasons why: the influx of foreign keepers, foreign coaches and how technically the modern keepers are not as good as in our generation. You might say they have to contend with balls that move faster and swerve more, but they moved in our time as well. But back then we had keepers who were technically better than they are today.

DAVID SEAMAN

I trained long enough with Shilts with England to know more than most about his abilities, his techniques and his training methods. In fact,

I learned an awful lot from him, alongside Chris Woods who also trained with myself and Shilts. The two main aspects of goalkeeping I learned from Shilts were his "shooting position" and his brilliant balance. It was these two aspects of his game play that made him able to stop so many shots on either side of him, without the need to second guess which side of the goal the striker was going to place his shot. Shilts had such brilliant balance that he could afford to wait until the forward committed himself to the shot.

Everyone has heard the stories about just how hard this guy would train. But it was much harder than anyone can imagine. I think you can only appreciate this by actually training with him. It was almost impossible to keep up with him in training. By the end of a session with him, you would be totally exhausted. It was impossible to train as hard as Shilts.

If I had to pick out my favourite Peter Shilton save, it would be the one-handed stop of the shot by Kenny Dalglish in England's game against the Scots. It's incredible to think he was wearing just those black cotton gloves back in those days, long before the technology developed into the current goalkeepers' gloves.

PAT JENNINGS

Peter Shilton... he's right up the with the best. It's a pleasure to write a tribute to him because he is a great goalkeeper. His record speaks for itself. I thought I was doing something exceptional – playing 119 internationals and playing into my 40s... but Peter Shilton, well, he was just unbelievable. Shilton was playing until he was 48 and winning a record 125 caps for England, having made his debut with Leicester at just sixteen. And to think that Leicester decided to get rid of the World Cup winning keeper Gordon Banks so that Peter could continue his amazing progression at that young age. Banks had won the World Cup! Moving on such a legend to nurture fresh talent says all you need to say about the young keeper that was coming through. Shilton proved you could play until such an age if you kept yourself fit.

I played against Peter's team when I came to Tottenham and was delighted to be in opposition to a player of such reputation. When I saw him in action I knew that his reputation was a deserved one. He had great agility, great hands – everything you need to be a great goalkeeper. Peter and I always had a chat after games, and I followed his career with interest. And what a great career – eventually winning back-to-back European Cups with Forest under Cloughie.

It's hard to make comparisons to modern day players. As everyone always says, you have to take into account that the pitches back then can't compare to the pitches of today which are immaculate. Despite all that has changed in the game, I can say with confidence that Shilts is as good as anyone.

There is that save against Scotland in 1973 that sticks in the mind. Watching it, we all thought he should go with his left hand, but he ended up saving the shot with his right. That save he made against Scotland was simply amazing. People might think it is unorthodox, but it is something that top goalkeepers will do if they are capable of doing it.

In our day we didn't have goalkeeping coaches, but Peter worked hard at his game. He would stay behind after sessions, asking strikers to hit shots at him. He was way ahead of his time and way ahead of everybody else at that stage.

JOE CORRIGAN

Peter Shilton! Where do you start? He can only be classed as one of the best goalkeepers in the world both in his day and in any era of the game. I was honoured to be amongst the three goalkeepers along with Shilts and Ray Clemence vying for the England jersey. And I learned so much from him – from his training regime, his technique – when you train and play with Shilts, you pick up knowledge from the best, and he was the very best. And I tried to put things I learned from him into my own training regime. When a man plays that many games for his country – a record number – put together with all his achievements, you cannot do anything other than put him right up there with the very best of all time.

From a personal point of view, I would say that Shilts is a true friend of mine. We were rivals on the pitch and teammates on the England squad. Although we were rivals at times, he taught me so much. Together with Clem (Ray Clemence), we were very much part of that old goalkeepers' union. For me, Shilts epitomised what goalkeeping was all about in our era – working hard, training hard and playing hard. Off the field he was always a true professional, but he is also quite a funny lad. He likes a joke, and he can take a joke. We were all very similar – professional, but we also enjoyed ourselves in our time off. Shilts was not an extrovert or a show-off. His sole purpose was to do his job well and he did. You can only admire what he did during his playing career. He's an amicable, very pleasant guy who likes a laugh and a joke and I am honoured to call him a friend of mine.

BOB WILSON

Peter Shilton was one of the greatest goalkeepers in the history of the game in this country. I can't give Shilts any greater praise, but there is no doubt that he merits it. There is an old saying in this game, "You only have the goalkeeper to beat." But in this case, if you were one to one with the keepers, you would then look up and say "Oh, shit. It's Shilton!"

My book, *You've Got to be Crazy*, features a chapter titled "The Magnificent Obsession". In it, I picked out only a handful of keepers to talk about and Shilts was one of them. Each of the keepers I selected was explored in a section of the chapter and each section opened with a quote from the individual. The one I picked out for Shilts was "It's an annoying part of me, something inside of me that won't tolerate second best. I don't want people to expect unbelievable things from me, but at the same time, I expect unbelievable things from myself." That explains the obsession goalkeepers have at the highest level. I had it. And so did any player wanting to reach the top in one of the loneliest positions in football – the one where you are the only individual in a team game. Shilts possessed that "magnificent obsession" with being the best. And reaching 125 caps for his country, where no other keeper has come remotely close in the 30 years since he achieved it, makes his story simply incredible. The fact that, as a young keeper at Leicester City he had so much ability and so much promise, that the club sold England football's beloved Gordon Banks, rated the best goalkeeper in the world at that time, to Stoke City to accommodate Shilts in their first team, says it all. Of course, that "magnificent obsession" began at an early age when he used to hang from the bannister at his childhood home with weights on his feet to stretch himself and make himself taller. That obsession was there from day one as he always believed he would make himself the greatest goalkeeper in the world. That obsession made him a perfectionist. All goalkeepers make mistakes irrespective of how good they are, but it's how they respond to them that makes the difference and nothing deflected Shilts.

I was working for the BBC during the World Cup in 1982. I recall being in the studios with the head of sport who was sure that Diego Maradona had scored a perfectly good goal against England in the quarter-finals. I told him it was a definite foul. I said, "Let's do a replay." That was ignored. A row broke out. "He (Shilton) was out jumped," I was told. "No, no, it was a foul," I insisted, "you have got to replay it." I was insistent. It was vital that we showed those watching that this was a foul. When we eventually played it back, it was a clear foul.

The best way I can sum up Peter Shilton's brilliance is what I wrote in my book in a tribute to that incredible career: "The only way Peter Shilton would admit to complete satisfaction is if his club side won the Football League Championship, the FA Cup and the Littlewoods Cup and if England won the World Cup or European Championship, and he didn't make any error of any description… all in the same season."

PETER SHILTON OBE, MBE: RECORDS, AWARDS & HONOURS, CAREER STATISTICS

RECORDS

Most competitive appearances ever in the world of football: an astonishing 1,390.

Shares the world record with Fabien Barthes of having ten clean sheets for goals conceded in seventeen matches in the history of World Cup games.

England's most capped player in men's football with an outstanding 125 caps.

Longest player in the history of English football to hold a cap record, currently standing at 30 years.

Record 1,005 league games played.

Made more appearances than any other England player at the old Wembley stadium: a record 52 appearances.

The oldest player to ever represent England at a World Cup.

IFFHS ranked Peter in 2000 as one of the top ten goalkeepers of the twentieth century.

AWARDS & HONOURS
Officer of the Order of the British Empire
Member of the Most Excellent Order of the British Empire

Club awards
Second Division 1970–71
FA Charity Shield 1971
First Division 1977–78
League Cup 1978–79
FA Charity Shield 1978
European Cup 1978–79 and 1979–80

International awards
Rous Cup 1986, 1988, 1989
FIFA World Cup fourth place 1990

Individual
ICO European Footballer of the Season 1979–80
PFA First Division Team of the Year: 1974–75, 1977–78, 1978–79, 1979–80, 1980–81, 1981–82, 1982–83, 1983–84, 1984–85, 1985–86
PFA Team of the Century 1977–1996
PFA Players 'Player of the year award' 1977–78
Nottingham Forest Player of the season 1981–82
Southampton Player of the season 1984–85, 1985–86
FWA Tribute Award 1991
English Football Hall of Fame 2002
Football League 100 Legends
Played for England at all levels Schoolboys, Youth, under-23s, Full International
Captained England fifteen times – more than any other goalkeeper

POSTSCRIPT BY STEPH SHILTON

AFTER HANGING UP THE GLOVES

After Peter hung up his gloves and boots he didn't walk away from the game. Peter is now regarded as one of the finest after-dinner football speakers in the UK. He also makes appearances and speeches all over the world. The locker room stories he has are endless because of the rare length of his extraordinary career, working with the biggest icons in English football history. Not only is Peter a highly successful speaker he also went on to become a motivational speaker. Many businesses have worked with him either as a guest speaker or as a brand endorser, including working as a brand ambassador for Seattle Sports where he took great interest in innovation. At 71 years old he is still very much on the football scene. He started playing in a football team at the tender age of nine, it's deep in his veins so it's not surprising for you to hear that 62 years later he's still supporting the industry he loves.

Peter remains working with the FA as one of their legendary visitors at events to help and support the industry. He also has remained as one of the FIFA all-time greats more recently supporting their think-tank sessions held in the UK. It's important to Peter that he maintains a close connection to the game.

Peter works with media outlets around the world including Sky Sports and makes regular TV appearances where he is valued for his commentary. But Peter has also consistently been in demand for his technical expertise and many view him as one of the greatest architects of the art of goalkeeping. We have to appreciate that Peter came from an era where training for goalkeepers didn't exist. This meant that many of the techniques and playing strategies he developed whilst playing have now formed the foundation for all modern-day goalkeeping training exercises.

Myself and Peter always try to visit his old clubs to watch his teams in our spare time. We rarely miss England matches at Wembley stadium. Every season he makes sure he returns back home to Leicester City, his birthplace and where it all began. We followed Leicester throughout that extraordinary season that saw them win the Premier League in 2016. Leicester City were complete outsiders, and nobody expected such a remarkable win, so it was an incredible moment for the City.

In October of 2018, both Peter and myself visited the King Power Stadium to watch a match against West Ham United. We left the Directors' Lounge not long after the crowds had dispersed and made our way to our car. We found the stadium car park emptying and relatively quiet. By coincidence another iconic Leicester goalkeeper, Kasper Schmeichel was leaving at the same time. Sadly, we were all witness to the horrific helicopter accident that took the lives of five people including the club's chairman, Vichai Srivaddhanaprabha. Peter and I saw the Chairman's helicopter hovering over the stadium. It then appeared to nosedive heading directly towards us. The pilot, we could see, was struggling to try and control the helicopter before it crashed. This was only around 60–80 feet from where we stood and roughly the same distance from Kasper. What we witnessed was horrific and I'm certain it will stay with us always. Leicester City went into deep grief at losing one the greatest and kindest club owners ever seen in this country. Vichai not only gave the club his full commitment, but he also cared deeply about the fans, and invested heavily in supporting the city of Leicester and local charities. His legacy and memory will never be forgotten. Pete and I will always have a deep affinity with Leicester City FC.

Peter is co-director along with myself of our company P&S.S.C Ltd (Peter & Steffi Shilton Consultancy Limited). We founded the company in 2017 and it provides promotional work and Peter's entire management. We have been extremely successful, and it means that the media and our clients have direct access to the company and to Peter instead of going via third parties.

Peter and I are also involved in several charities and we try to support a minimum of six events every year. We have personally raised thousands of pounds for various charities, including Haven House Children's Hospice and the St. Helena Hospice, Colchester. In October 2019, on Mental Health Awareness day we raised £15,000 in one evening for the charity Mind at a gala event at Colchester United Stadium. We are both ambassadors for The Essex Disabled Sports Foundation which, along with The President's Sporting Club have raised well over £2.5 million which has been used for special educational need schools and organisations to provide sporting equipment, facilities and opportunities for disabled children and those with special needs. The charity sponsored young swimmer Helen Thompson who won the world record championship for the 100m individual medley at the Down Syndrome Championship.

Peter directed his own video series named *Shilton's Secrets: The Art of Goalkeeping*, which showcases the goalkeeping techniques that he developed and perfected over his long and illustrious career. It examines fourteen different techniques that should be used by a goalkeeper in his training exercises. It's Peter's way of ensuring the techniques he personally developed can remain as part of his career legacy.

Peter Shilton is undoubtedly one of the greatest goalkeepers in the history of football, his records and achievements are remarkable. Peter's legacy will remain always in the history and at the heart of England's three lions.

Steph xx

THE REFEREE'S ROOM

POSTSCRIPT 1 – THE RT. HON SIR IAIN DUNCAN SMITH, MP

The significant impact which gambling has had on Peter's life is, tragically, an experience shared by far too many. Gambling has been allowed to proliferate in this country and we simply do not have the right regulations in place to prevent harm and the right treatment systems in place to support people. We need to be inspired by Peter and Steph's courage and ensure that our gambling laws are properly reformed and provide the protection that we all deserve and the most vulnerable desperately need.

POSTSCRIPT 2 – CHARLES RITCHIE

Jack Ritchie (28/12/92 – 22/11/17)

Our son Jack was born in December 1992. Peter Shilton may have ended his international playing career more than two years before but his stature and reputation in the game was such that Peter was one of Jack's earliest childhood footballing heroes. Jack's first engagement and fascination with football was as a goalkeeper and, like all little boys who love their football, he did his homework. He knew his history. He became a mine of information about football, and Peter Shilton loomed large.

Jack loved football from a very early age. I recall watching the Euro '96 tournament with him when he was just three years old. Even then he knew the players' names and followed with a fascination and attention way beyond his years.

But he didn't just watch, he loved playing – he was forever kicking a football about in the garden on his own while loudly narrating the commentary or playing with friends. And then, at junior school, he got involved in his first team games – playing in goal for Ecclesall Rangers. He shared goalkeeping duties with his friend Greg: shades of the Shilton/Clemence era sharing England duties? And he was good. Always big for his age, he was a commanding presence in goal and had good positional sense. And he was a good shot-stopper. His commitment knew no bounds: once playing on with a fractured wrist incurred in saving a penalty.

From a young age he'd make up imaginary clubs, leagues and competitions. His attention to detail was extraordinary. Each "club" had their own kit and named players. And tournaments would be played out over days. All of that took on another dimension when he was old enough for the FIFA series of computer football games. His knowledge of European clubs and footballers from around the world soon surpassed mine. He grasped an astonishing level of detail about all the clubs and players. It all seemed so natural and harmless… back then.

And he always enjoyed watching football. Having flirted with Manchester United as a little boy – they were winning everything at the time – he soon developed a strong allegiance to his local club, Sheffield United. The trophies weren't as plentiful, but he understood that football wasn't just about silverware. It was about the shared passion with your mates; the peaks and troughs; the belonging.

He never lost his love of football. As he grew older, he played for many teams – often playing for several at the same time. He would always seek out a game and a team wherever he was. At university he played for the Chemistry Society team… despite studying for a history degree! When he was out volunteering in Kenya in 2017, he organised a football match that ended up with the volunteers taking on a team of 30 or 40 young people from the local village.

Tragically, something else entered Jack's life when he was just seventeen. Gambling took a bright, normal, happy, popular seventeen-year-old who was enjoying life and had a great future ahead of him and killed him before he was 25. Like so many of his generation, Jack came across gambling as an apparently harmless and fun activity. That was how it was portrayed then and, shamefully, that is still how the gambling industry tries to portray it today.

Jack began gambling during his lunchtime at school. He used to go to the local bookies with a group of his schoolmates to play the, now infamous, Fixed Odds Betting Terminals (FOBTs). A big group of schoolboys, never challenged about their age were gambling their dinner money every day. Most days they'd lose and go hungry but some days there would be an extra portion of chips. But Jack was the unlucky one, because very early on he won big. Twice. One lunchtime he won £500 in successive spins. So, as a seventeen-year-old schoolboy, he went to school with a fiver in his pocket and came back with £1,000. Of course, we didn't know about any of this at the time.

About a year later when he told us what had happened – of course by then he'd lost that £1000 as well as some other money that his grandmother had given him – we didn't understand the seriousness of what Jack was facing. *He* didn't know. We thought that it was just a "phase" he was going through; he was just a teenage boy and we said to ourselves that he'd "grow out of it". We now understand that, by the time we found out, Jack probably already had a deep and complex condition. And we also didn't know about the high suicide risk around these kinds of addictions. We didn't know that gambling kills. If we had learned that he was shooting up heroin, we would have acted so differently. His friends would have. His school would have. His doctor would have. Jack would have. But we were all ignorant. We know now that we were deliberately kept ignorant. After all, gambling was "just a bit of fun": the government wouldn't allow such a dangerous product on the high street with no health warnings.

We now know that some gambling products, like the FOBTs and the same products which are now freely available on your mobile phone, are highly toxic and addictive. FOBTs have addiction/at risk rates of over 50 per cent: you are more likely to be seriously harmed by them than not. And the damage is permanent. It is not the money that you lose, it is what gambling does to your brain, to your mental health. It is the very real and high risk to your life. People with a gambling disorder are over fifteen times more likely to take their own lives than the general population. Over ten per cent of suicides are linked to gambling: that

185

is over 600 deaths per year in the UK alone. A six-year-old knows that smoking kills; how many people know that gambling kills?

We now know that research shows a very high correlation between a big early win and the development of gambling disorder. And let's be clear, gambling disorder is not just a "bad habit", it is a serious psychiatric condition. In 2013 it was classified as a behavioural disorder alongside alcohol and drug addiction. It is a serious, complex addiction. Gambling alters your brain permanently and young brains being particularly vulnerable.

Jack struggled with the addiction for seven years. We worked with him; self-excluding from local bookies; buying gambling blocking software for his phone and computer. He spoke to his GP about it and had sessions of group and individual therapy. He could be free of gambling for weeks and months at a time, but he would always be dragged back in… The barrage of advertising and direct offers of free bets and money was constant and impossible to avoid.

Jack never lost huge amounts of money. He died with an overdraft of £1,500 and a half paid off bank loan of £2,000. But it was clear from his suicide note that it was gambling that had killed him. He felt that he would never be free of it, that it would always drag him back in. Gambling had ruined Jack's mental health. He took his own life in November 2017, just one month short of his 25th birthday.

Soon after Jack died, we were introduced to another family in Sheffield who had lost their 25-year-old son just six months before and a family in the South West who had lost their son a month before Jack. Both were suicides caused by gambling: bright, happy, outgoing young men with no other problems in life. They were killed by gambling – 100 per cent.

That was the start of Gambling with Lives. We realised that we were not on our own, so we set out to find and contact other families. After a few weeks of trawling local newspaper stories, contacting coroners and suicide bereavement support groups, we had identified around 40 gambling related suicides. Many of the families were still too distraught to speak or become involved. Many felt that they had to keep quiet for a variety of personal and cultural issues.

But a core group of ten families met up in Birmingham in August 2018. And, as we told each other our stories, we came to realise that all of the young people we had lost were so similar – bright, normal, happy and popular young folk from happy families and with great futures ahead of them. All destroyed by gambling.

We read and collated the international research and estimated that there were between 250 and 650 gambling related suicides every year in the UK – five to ten per cent of all suicides. Introducing suicide to the debate on gambling regulation has perhaps been our greatest public achievement: consideration of the scale of suicides and the fact that this is happening to ordinary young people cannot be ignored whenever gambling is discussed today.

So, for the past two and half years Gambling with Lives has been working hard to combat the appalling harms caused by gambling. One side of the work has focused on supporting families who have been bereaved by gambling suicides. This has been enormously powerful and provides the impetus to keep going to prevent other families ever being devastated like we have.

The other side has involved awareness raising and campaigning for tougher gambling regulation. We have met Ministers and MPs from across the political spectrum and given evidence to the House of Lords, the Gambling Related Harms All-Party Parliamentary Group and the Gambling Commission; spoken with officials from the regulator and gambling charities. We have met with treatment specialists and international researchers. We've presented at conferences and events and held two events in the Houses of Parliament which were attended by dozens of MPs and Lords and one in Stormont which helped to launch the review of gambling in Northern Ireland. I've lost count of the number of TV, radio and press interviews that we've done in this country and abroad. We've even spoken to people working in the gambling industry.

Perhaps most importantly we have met dozens of people who are in recovery from gambling disorder. And what an incredible bunch of people they are – sharp, intelligent, thoughtful people who could not be more different from the image of an addict. They are people who absolutely put a lie to the myth about gambling disorder being about a small number of flawed individuals: these are bright people who were high achievers with outgoing personalities, witty, personable… people who you would want on your side, in your team.

Which brings me to the call that we got, out of the blue, in January 2020 from Steph Shilton. She'd seen the Gambling with Lives website and wanted to speak. We had a long talk with her over the phone. She told us about Pete's gambling addiction and that, as a couple, they wanted to do something public to alert people to the serious dangers of gambling.

I had read somewhere about Pete's problems in the past but had no idea of the details covered in this book. I was full of admiration for their bold decision. We had long recognised that gambling was a major problem within professional football and had tried to engage with many of the former players who were now acting as celebrity "ambassadors" for gambling companies. But there was a staggering lack of understanding (deliberate or otherwise) of what gambling was like today – industrialised electronic gambling available 24/7 on your mobile with constant marketing, free bets and "spins" for everyone, and VIP schemes offering trips, gifts and thousands of pounds for those who lost the most… whether they could afford it or not. And no one understood the reality of addiction.

Steph organised for me to speak with Pete before he was due to meet the Minister of Sport to discuss football and gambling. At first, it was a strange conversation for me. I was old enough to have seen Pete in his prime and could never decide whether he or Gordon Banks ranked higher! And I knew that the young Jack would have been overawed and speechless. But quite quickly we were speaking as two people whose lives had been torn apart by gambling. He told me something of his story with the openness of someone who had finally understood what had happened to him and was obviously totally supported by his wife. It was clear that Steph was a real tower of strength for him and that the two of them were determined to do everything that they could to get change.

Pete's story was very different to Jack's. The scale of their financial losses were absolutely miles apart. But it was clear that both of them had begun gambling with no idea that it was so dangerous and that it posed a severe risk to mental health. It was also clear that both had been abused by an industry which was out of control and had no purpose other than extracting as much money as quickly as possible from its customers. It is a business model built on addiction with no concern about the well-being of individuals. It was brutal. The legendary Peter Shilton had been exploited as ruthlessly as Jack Ritchie from Sheffield.

It was clearly a big decision for Pete and Steph to go public about his addiction. But, like the Gambling with Lives families, they both recognised that changes to gambling and gambling regulation were needed to stop the appalling harms which are occurring every day. They have played a very astute game, using Pete's celebrity and the great warmth and affection that the British public has for him. And their generosity to Gambling with Lives has been remarkable: they kindly donated their fees for their early TV appearances and press to the charity.

We know that we will continue to work with them – sharing information and collaborating wherever we can. Always speaking out and raising awareness and trying to make sure that no one else has to suffer in the ways that we have. So, thank you both, Pete and Steph. All power to you and we'll celebrate with you both when, together, we achieve those changes that are needed.

POSTSCRIPT 3 – CAROLYN HARRIS, Member of Parliament for Swansea East; Parliamentary Private Secretary to the Leader of the Opposition, Sir Keir Starmer; Chair of the All-Party Parliamentary Group on Gambling-Related Harm.

Peter and Steph should be applauded for their campaign. I have been really impressed that someone as world famous as Peter Shilton has stood up and been brave enough to use his dreadful experiences for so much good. It must have been very difficult to open up, much more difficult when you are in the limelight to go up front and have people challenge you, criticise you, and make negative from so much of the positive you are trying to do.

Also, not everyone has got a Steph in their lives to help them through such a terrible addiction. Instead, a lot of people have to face it alone. It can ruin their lives, badly affect and even destroy their families. It can lead, in some cases, to sufferers breaking the law to feed their addiction and ending up in jail. And, in far too many cases, it can lead to sufferers taking their own lives. Peter and Steph have survived one of the worst experiences any couple could face together – a gambling addiction. It is far worse than most people can imagine, it can suck the life out of you and your family, and it can change your attitude to life.

I am so glad that Steph was there for Peter, and I am sure that this book has told a story that will be an eye-opener for those who have never been touched by the addiction of gambling. I hope it will also be a blessing for those who are affected, and who believe there is no way out. I hope that, in Peter and Steph's story, they can see that there is a way out. Everybody out there suffering from this dreadful addiction can find solace from Peter and Steph's story, see how they survived it and how you too can survive it.

There are growing numbers of those affected by, and indeed, addicted to gambling, far too many. The help that they need can in part come from those in power who can challenge the gambling industry practices and change legislation. I met Peter and Steph and took them to the House of Commons to meet Sir Iain Duncan Smith as I know how much this issue means to them both, and how much they are doing to help us with our campaign to make changes to the law. Those changes are vitally important.

In 2016 I set up an All-Party Group to look into Fixed Odds Betting Terminals, and I am delighted to say that this was instrumental in bringing down the stakes on those gambling machines from £100 every twenty seconds to a stake of £2. It was clear that allowing people to gamble such high stakes on machines that were so addictive was anti-social. It had become increasingly obvious it needed to be resolved despite all the barriers to change there were, not just the gambling industry, but also the UK Treasury who were making a fortune in tax.

That was an important battle to win, but it became clear there was another equally important battle ahead, and that is to tackle online gambling addiction and sports betting which has mushroomed over the years to become an epidemic of worrying proportions. My involvement with the All-Party Group on slot machines grew organically and I became involved with the All-Party Group on Gambling Related Harm, which put the spotlight on this new and worrying form of gambling addiction. I receive, every single day, at least ten to fifteen emails or messages from somebody who is trapped by online gambling addiction.

I should at this point stop and emphasise that I am in no way anti-gambling. I am more than delighted for the people who enjoy a little flutter on their weekly bingo, or enjoy betting, but so long as it is within their means and not because they are being exploited by the aggressive marketing and advertising from the betting industry that lures them into a life of intolerable addiction. If you can't walk away from placing a bet then, in all probability, you have become a victim of this exploitation. This is something we have to stand up against, and that's why it is so important that we can count on people such as Peter and Steph.

It is no exaggeration in stating that the scandal here is that the gambling industry grooms people. You only have to look at the VIP accounts where you have to spend £1,500 per week to qualify, which they are granting to members who only earn £400 per week. To fuel that gambling addiction people will get into debt or even to crime and often end up in jail. Many will resort to taking their own lives as the only way out. I have case studies coming out of my ears of such cases. It is awful. Just awful. Something has to be done, and something *is* being done.

The emphasis for me is the harm it is doing to children and how early in a child's development they can become hooked on gambling. It is *staggeringly* young. It is simply appalling and heartbreaking.

We know many football clubs rely heavily on income from the gambling industry and especially the lower league clubs who are suffering the devastating effects of the Covid 19 pandemic, which has robbed them of the lifeblood of their industry, the paying customers. I have become aware of a three-year-old who has named his teddy bear "Betway" because he has seen the name Betway on the front of his team's football shirt. In October 2020, front page of the *Sunday People* newspaper exposed just how many children are enticed by gambling and how much children are spending. It is frightening just how many of these kids are becoming addicts.

But there is going to be change, with the National Audit Office reviewing the government's plans for reform and for new legislation, made clear in their manifesto. The Lords set up their own review of the gambling industry and its effects on addiction, to which the government are obliged to respond. The Lords report on gambling regulation called for "urgent action." The House of Lords Gambling Select Committee's report "Gambling Harm – Time for Action" took over a year to compile and the results did not make comfortable reading for the industry, the regulator and the government. On its launch, Committee Chair Lord Grade of Yarmouth said: "Urgent action by the Government is required. Lax regulation of the gambling industry must be replaced by a more robust and focused regime which prioritises the welfare of gamblers ahead of industry profits. Addiction is a health problem which should be treated by the NHS and paid for by gambling industry profits. The government must impose a mandatory levy on the industry. The more harmful a gambling product is, the higher the levy the operator should pay."

I know Michael Grade, and the report is indeed something that has moved the agenda forward. It made 66 recommendations including specifically on gambling: the creation of a statutory independent Gambling Ombudsman Service, a ban on "bet to view" streaming contracts, and more supervision from the regulator on "single manning" (a single member of staff only) in licenced betting offices. On gaming, all new games should be tested for harm indicators before launch. The speed of online games matched with speed of land-based equivalents and online games get categorised like land-based ones with stake restrictions. There was also the call for a ban on sports teams' kit sponsorship and venue advertising for gambling companies with an exemption only for horse racing and greyhounds. The plan to ban shirt advertising is something dear to my heart, and is something I have been working on, even though there will be an exemption until 2023 for non-Premier League football and other sports. There is also independent research into links between advertising and gambling-related harm.

I contacted Trevor Birch, a vastly experienced and knowledgeable football administrator, who aided Ken Bates with the Roman Abramovich takeover at Chelsea, whilst he was chairman at Swansea FC. I convinced him that the UBet advertising of the Chinese betting company should be removed from the front of their shirts, and he agreed. Trevor is now at Spurs and I would like him to do the same there.

The issue is that while other companies would offer a Championship club say £1 million for front of shirt advertising, the betting companies would blow that out of the water by offering £5 million. A club can find it difficult to resist, certainly in these troubled times, when so many clubs are threatened with going out of business, and struggling companies are even less likely to be able to compete with the vast amounts betting companies have at their disposal for this kind of aggressive advertising. Naturally, the Premier League are terrified about their clubs losing revenue and are doing as much as they can to delay the process, but they won't prevent the new legislation. The EFL issued a statement saying they "continue to have an open and regular dialogue with all relevant stakeholders – including the Government – regarding football's ongoing relationship with the gambling industry to ensure its partnerships are activated in a responsible fashion." But we all know that they are protecting their sources of income. The Football League added: "The association between football and the gambling sector is long-standing, with a collaborative, evidence-based approach to preventing gambling harms of much greater benefit than that of a blanket ban of any kind. Through a highly visible awareness and education campaign, the EFL and Sky Bet work together to promote responsible gambling, with players from all three divisions wearing sleeve badges to encourage supporters to consider how they gamble and 70 per cent of the sponsor's match day inventory dedicated to safer gambling messaging." But whilst it's pretty easy to see the Sky Bet logo on the sleeve badges, their message about betting responsibly is pretty hard to read.

The League pointed out that over £40 million a season is paid by the betting industry, either centrally to the League and or to its clubs. They openly admit "the significant contribution betting companies make to the ongoing financial sustainability of professional football at all levels is as important now as it has ever been, particularly given the ongoing impact of the Covid 19 pandemic which is leaving many of our clubs living on a financial knife edge."

They also point out that the clubs contribute almost £500 million annually to the Exchequer but has had "its core income stream of ticket sales turned off indefinitely without any indication of a roadmap that will allow the safe return of supporters to stadiums, despite other sectors being able to welcome people through their doors." Therefore, they conclude: "Our approach in respect of gambling sponsorship is under constant review and the League will also contribute to any call for evidence by the Government as we seek to protect an important and vital income stream for our membership in a time of financial crisis." Well, there it is. A clear public confession that their prime motivation is protecting the money streams to their clubs, and indeed to themselves. But make no mistake the day of reckoning is upon the football industry in terms of curbing sports sponsorship and shirt advertising.

There are numerous other measures we need in place such as raising the minimum age for the National Lottery, any online gambling and even the seaside arcade cash machine bandits from sixteen to eighteen.

Certainly, when it comes to football and its relationship with gambling, the voice of the likes of Peter and Steph Shilton need to be heard. Findings have shown that footballers are three times more likely to become gambling addicts. They too can be fragile and vulnerable like the rest of us, if they cannot pull back from what is a slippery slope to addiction and all that entails. Pete and Steph's voices have been heard through this book which will not just be a record of their own battle against gambling addiction but a tool to help others similarly affected and not just elite sportsmen and footballers but ordinary people as well.

But the biggest worry, the gravest concern, is that this country is creating a new generation of gambling addicts. The most at risk are children and starting from an incredibly young age. This cannot be ignored and needs to be acted on. The damage has already been done – damage beyond belief – but it has to stop, and we are determined that it will stop. Peter and Steph Shilton have been effective and active campaigners, and so many charity groups have emerged to support action, such as Gambling with Lives, Big Step, GambleAware, with so much social media activity, and different groups emerging with the same common aim, and that needs to be applauded.

POSTSCRIPT 4 – BRIAN CHAPPELL, Justice for Punters

Justice for Punters (J4P) was set up five years ago by volunteers who knew that the gambling industry didn't trade fairly or safely even after the implementation of the UK's Gambling Act (2005). They have collected case and other evidence and campaigned for improvements ever since. They all give their time freely and fund J4P themselves. There are many conflicts of financial interest within the gambling industry, J4P staunchly avoids this.

The Modern Day Gambling Industry

In the year 2008–09 the gross gambling yield (the amount lost by gamblers) in the UK was £8.4 billion. In 2018–19 it was £14.3 billion.

This means the amount lost has increased by 70 per cent in the last decade.

Inflation during this period amounted to 31 per cent and UK average weekly earnings increased by 22.2 per cent. Clearly, people on average UK weekly earnings are worse off now than in 2009, but at the same time gambling losses have massively increased. Also clear, is that the gambling industry is doing extremely well. This success is hardly surprising when people are now able to carry a casino in their pocket in the form of their mobile phone.

It is important to recognise that the modern gambling industry isn't what it appears to be. It is sold as being another form of safe entertainment – fun if you like, a chance for all to win money 24/7. This is especially so, if you think you really understand the risks and the dangers. The industry gives punters warnings after all. "Don't be silly. Bet savvy" was a recent betting company advert slogan.

If you have a family member who is gambling regularly, they are certainly losing money. How do we know this? It's simple really. The modern, corporate-dominated gambling industry only trades with people who lose. If a customer starts regularly winning either because they are particularly skilled or through sheer luck, they will effectively be banned from gambling by what are called stake restrictions. So, a particularly successful punter will try to place a £10 bet and they will be offered just 23p, 10p or even 1p. Anyone gambling who is not being offered these kind of stake restrictions is losing money overall by gambling.

These losses may be affordable for some wealthy customers. The ultimate gambling company service for extracting more money is VIP status for customers they have identified as good sources of cash. The VIP status will include invitations to sporting events, special deals on free bets or free spins. All of these are aimed at increasing the amount and the frequency of the customer's gambling. Gambling companies do not provide free lunches. But the gambling industry has become superb at extracting more money from every customer – not just the wealthier ones – by offering a myriad of opportunities to gamble, new, more immersive gambling products and faster ways to gamble. In betting shops now, there is an event at least every 60 seconds to gamble on. Perhaps the most sinister thing that the companies do is sophisticated online customer profiling. Sucked in by all these lures, the punter may eventually find they go on to lose money that should be paying their rent, a mortgage or even their food bills.

A Myriad of Opportunities to Gamble

If you want a chance to win back your losses, the gambling industry is now there for you 24/7. Until recently, it was possible to spin a slot game more than once a second. These games can be played at stakes of £100, £200 and £400 per spin. There are many potential winning lines, flashing lights, music reinforced "wins" – some which are often losses disguised as wins, that is a win which is less than the total staked. Everything is designed to speed up play in a confusing way. You have to be immersed to know what is going on. These products need to be tested for safety. In the UK some companies abide by a new rule that dictates there must be 2.5 seconds between spins. Any change is to be welcomed, but 2.5 seconds? Really? Will it be effective? There has to be doubt.

People who have a gambling disorder often talk about being "in the zone". They often see gambling as a way to block out other things in their life they don't wish to think about. Therefore being "in the zone" is important to them. Gambling industry executives are well aware of this, so you'd think they'd design products that gave customers a chance to think, a chance to reflect and an option to leave "the zone". Nothing of the sort, the gambling industry has used rogue psychologists to design products that are immersive and highly addictive. And the industry really like it if they can encourage customers to bet on things they're likely to know nothing about or have a guaranteed "in-house" profit.

When people approach companies with concerns about loved ones the gambling industry will tell them it is their fault and that they need some self-control. The gambling industry needs to provide more safeguards and protection for their customers and recognise that providing this myriad of 24/7 gambling opportunities could be potentially harmful.

Sophisticated Online Customer Profiling

Many people aren't aware that, from the moment you land on the home page of a gambling website, you are being profiled. The main aims are to ensure you aren't winning for too long using skill and to target marketing that will appeal to you if you lose and encourage you to gamble more frequently.

All new customers are rapidly rated using algorithms that dictate how much that person can stake and on what. If you lose betting on a football match, you will be targeted with promotions about betting on football. The same for horse racing, greyhound racing and any sport you wish to choose. If you show signs of a successful winning streak on a sport your stake will be restricted and if you still keep winning that stake restriction may go down to 1p or even nil.

Historically and still today gambling companies tend not to complete affordability checks until the damage is done. Justice for Punters regularly sees cases where losses of thousands per month were never checked. What proportion of the UK's population have enough disposable income to lose thousands per month? That's the problem in a nutshell, but the UK government, its regulator and the gambling companies have failed to address this and implement sensible rules and regulations.

The modern gambling industry does provide entertainment, but it is also ruthless. At Justice for Punters we describe their business model as "ban or bankrupt". As a punter, you cannot win.

POSTSCRIPT 5 – MATT GASKELL, C.Psychol AFBPsS, Consultant Psychologist & Clinical Lead, NHS Northern Gambling Service

The Need for Gambling Reform

The publication of this important book coincides with the expansion of specialist gambling treatment clinics by the National Health Service (NHS). By 2023/24 there will be fifteen clinics across England. The new ones will complement the existing ones in London (The National Problem Gambling Clinic), and Leeds, Manchester and Sunderland (which form The NHS Northern Gambling Service). In addition to providing treatment for the gambler, they also offer specific help for those affected by a loved one's gambling addiction. So, whether you find yourself in Peter's shoes, or Steph's shoes, there is specialist help on the

NHS. We also have the UK's first NHS gambling treatment clinic for children from the age of thirteen, based in London.

These clinics would not have existed were it not for our liberal gambling laws. When I was growing up, gambling, in general, was a low-profile activity. Betting shop windows were blacked out, there was no advertising, and online gambling was unheard of. As a mad football fan, betting wasn't on the radar of my peer group. We could just focus on our love of the game. In retrospect I was fortunate to grow up at that time.

Gambling addiction existed before the 2005 Gambling Act, as Peter's story demonstrates, but the change in law has opened the floodgates and our society is reaping the consequences. This is the era of deregulation and the expansion of commercial gambling worldwide. It was particularly unfortunate timing, as the new laws came in before smartphones, laptops and tablets. Now you have a super casino in your pocket, in your workplace, at university and in your own home, with access 24 hours a day. If you are attracted to gambling, it is all too easy to form a habit. Discontinuous forms of gambling (like the outcome of a football match, horse race or National Lottery) have been overtaken by continuous, high speed gambling products and events, often played in isolation online (such as slot machines, roulette, or in-play sports betting). These carefully designed products and ways of gambling are both revenue generating and habit forming. They deliver both the anticipation and excitement of a win, as well as an escape from everyday life. Advertising, sponsorship and the promotion of gambling is ubiquitous in our lives. No surprise given an annual advertising budget of £1.5bn. Egregious VIP schemes provide free bets, free money and other rewards to many who have already lost themselves to gambling addiction. Our high streets have been transformed by the clustering of bookmakers, particularly in our more deprived communities.

Gambling has been carefully reframed from being a potential source of crime, to a fun entertaining leisure pursuit, endorsed by celebrities and sports stars. We consistently see and hear "When the fun stops, stop" and "Gamble responsibly". The burden of responsibility is placed upon the individual gambler, and not the products or practices of the gambling industry, with the result that many don't seek help for the deep shame this causes. The truth, in my view, is more complex. We all live in this commercial world; the environment and influences around us shaping our attitudes and behaviour.

Gambling is now hand in glove with football, our nation's favourite sport, as well as others such as snooker, rugby league, and darts. Whilst, of course, many people can bet without it causing impairment to their life, the commercial gambling environment we live in, and the lack of protection for consumers, leaves a largely hidden trail of devastation for individuals, families and communities up and down the land. In addition to the lack of protection and regulation, the harm is being done without any public health messaging to warn of the dangers of what some are calling the "gamblification" of our lives.

In 2010 the last British Gambling Prevalence Survey estimated there were 450,000 adults with a gambling addiction. By 2020 a YouGov survey estimated this number was 1.4 million. Whilst these are just estimates, these results won't come as a shock to those of us who have observed the proliferation of gambling. This estimate doesn't include the millions "at risk" of a gambling addiction, nor all those who could lose all their rent money or money to feed their family, in one gambling episode. This would never show up on such surveys. As Steph's account very ably demonstrates, gambling also deeply affects loved ones, families and friends. An average of five to ten people are affected by someone else's gambling addiction. Gambling amongst children occurs more frequently than smoking, drinking or taking drugs, and between 2014 and 2016 gambling addiction amongst children aged eleven to sixteen quadrupled, according to The Gambling Commission. When you put all of this together we have a significant public health concern on our hands. Peter and Steph's book coincides with the review of our gambling legislation. And change can't come soon enough. The tide is turning thanks to brave accounts like Pete's and Steph's, and the families from the charity Gambling with Lives who have lost their cherished children to gambling-related suicide. I think we will look back on this period with some horror, just as we do when we look back to the days when the many were smoking in pubs, cars and on aeroplanes.

The best thing we can do is to change our laws, have tougher regulation and better protect our kids and the next generation. However, for those whose gambling becomes excessive or for those who get lost in the fog of a gambling addiction, help is at hand.

Face-to-Face Gambling Treatment for Individuals and Families
Attending a treatment service can seem a daunting prospect for some. However, meeting with specialists who understand addiction and peers who are also recovering from gambling problems can be transformative and empowering. The best therapy available is cognitive-behavioural therapy, so check to see that this is provided. Most services also offer access to people with lived experience of gambling problems, who act as role models and mentors.

Good treatment will help you develop a positive bond with a therapist, strengthen your motivation and confidence to stop gambling, block opportunities and access to gamble, avoid or cope with cravings and high-risk situations, change your gambling thoughts, change your behaviour and routines, access new rewarding ways to live your life, develop positive bonds with family and friends and enlist their support, practice new skills, and learn to live to your potential. Some services, such as the NHS clinics, can also provide specialist mental health and well-being support.

For family members, treatment and support is also available. This tends to focus on coping with the challenges and stress of dealing with a loved one's addiction.

POSTSCRIPT 6 – LINDA UDALL and HARRY HARRIS
We feel incredibly privileged to have been able to support both Peter and Steph in the writing of this book – their words literally came from their hearts. This extraordinary couple had to face their darkest moments together and revisit those painful memories through these pages. In *Saved* they have both laid bare their heart-wrenching experience of gambling addiction for the first time. It is a story that unfolds from both the addict and the victim's perspective. This is an emotionally honest and revealing book. The words are their own and come from their very hearts. Their voices and their true story.

Working with them as part of the team for many, many hours has truly been an honour and being part of their journey has been fascinating. We have witnessed first-hand how passionate they are about bringing that much needed change to the gambling industry. During our time with Peter and Steph, we learnt so much about the condition and the gambling industry that we had no prior knowledge of before – it certainly has been an eye-opener. We finished the project with a completely different view of gambling addiction and we're sure all those that read this book will do the same.

Pete and Steph are a force to be reckoned with. Their strength and the love between them means they have a bond that is unbreakable. We know they will accomplish everything they set out to do.

Cheers to you both, Mr and Mrs S.

STEPH'S WEDDING DAY POEM TO PETE, 10TH DECEMBER 2016

We would like to dedicate these words that Steph wrote to Pete to you all.

TO MISTER FROM YOUR TITCH

Look back Mister, on the night that we met
When fate sealed us together and our hearts were set

We trusted each other and we shared all
We built our tower, that now stands strong and tall

As long as we have forever, my kind Sir
I will be your lady at your side
I will be your friend, your companion and your guide

As long as I live and as long as you care
I will do anything for you, I will go anywhere

We've braved life's mountains, as we have strived together
There are no storms we cannot weather

I will bring you the sunshine, as we comfort each other's fears
I will continue to gather rainbows and chase away tears

We're starting our new journey, a new exciting life
As you take my small hand and name me your wife

As long as we have forever, my love, I will always be true
As long as we have forever, my Sir, I will love only you

SUPPORT FOR GAMBLING PROBLEMS

Not everyone will want, or need, formal gambling treatment. Recognising you have a problem, talking to loved ones and receiving their support is often the best first step you can take. Someone you trust could temporarily manage your money until you feel free of gambling cravings.

There are additional measures you can take, which we call "stimulus control". For example, you can switch on a "gambling transaction block" on your mobile banking app. These are available via high street banks such as Barclays, HSBC, Halifax and Lloyds. Typically, if you change your mind, there is a 24–72 hour wait before you can gamble, which is very useful when the desire to gamble strikes. Online banks such as Monzo and Starling Bank, are notably showing the way by launching in-app gambling blocks in 2018.

You can also use blocking software on all your devices that will prevent access to gambling websites.

A recommended one is **Gamban**, which can be found at **www. gamban.com**.

You can self-exclude on a specific gambling operator website, but the best thing would be to self-exclude from all licensed operators in one go, using **Gamstop**, which is available free at **www.gamstop.co.uk**.

There are schemes available to self-exclude from more than one bookmaker in your area via **0800 294 2060**, bingo venues via **www. bingo-association.co.uk/self-exclusion**, or **0203 409 2047**, and arcades and adult gaming centres via **www.bacta.org.uk/self-exclusion.**

There is also online support for gambling problems via **Gambling Therapy** at **www.gamblingtherapy.org/en**. This provides practical and emotional support and is available in a number of different languages.

Online live chat, message forums and support are also available via the national gambling charity **GamCare** at **www.gamcare.org.uk**. They also operate the **National Gambling Helpline** on **0808 8020 133** and have access to local counselling provision.

For specific support to manage debt then you can contact **Step Change** via **www.stepchange.org**, **Money Advice Service** via **www.moneyadviceservice.org.uk** as well as **Citizens Advice Bureau** on **www.citizensadvice.org.uk**, and **www.nationaldebtline.org**.

NHS Northern Gambling Service (covering the north of England with clinics in Manchester, Leeds, and Sunderland) on **0300 300 1490** or via **www.leedsandyorkpft.nhs.uk/our-services/northern-gambling-service/**. Virtual consultations are also available.

NHS National Problem Gambling Clinic (covers Southern England) on **020 7381 7722** or via

www.cnwl.nhs.uk/services/mental-health-services/addictions-and-substance-misuse/national-problem-gambling-clinic. Virtual consultations are also available.

Residential treatment via **Gordon Moody Association** in the Midlands & South London: **www.gordonmoody.org.uk**.

Support via **The Primary Care Gambling Service** in London on **0300 0300 111**.

Gamblers Anonymous: **www.gamblersanonymous.org.uk**.

Gamblers Anonymous Scotland: **www.gascotland.org**.

Gam-Anon (support for family members): **www.gamanon.org.uk**.

Gamfam (support for family members): **www.gamfam.co.uk**.

Samaritans: **www.samaritans.org** or by phone: **116 123**.

Peter & Steffi Shilton Consultancy Ltd: **steffi.shilton@yahoo.com**